Back *to* Life

With 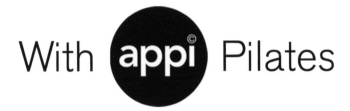 Pilates

A Six-Week Programme

TO REFINE, TONE AND STRENGTHEN YOUR BODY

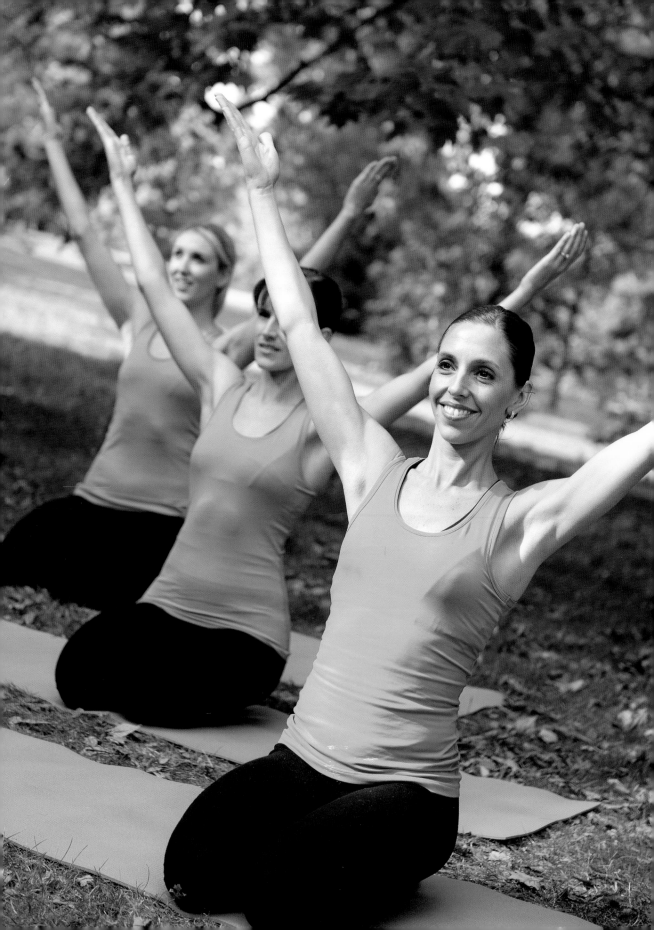

Back *to* Life

With 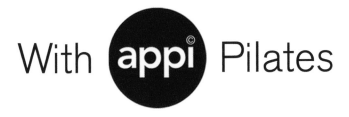 Pilates

A Six-Week Programme
TO REFINE, TONE AND STRENGTHEN YOUR BODY

To Jasmine and Xavier,
our angels and young Pilates devotees

First published in Great Britain in 2011 by APPI Health Group Ltd

TEXT © Elisa and Glenn Withers

PHOTOGRAPHY © Malin Christenson and Laurent Liotardo

The right of Elisa Withers and Glenn Withers to be identified as the Authors of the Work has been asserted by them in accordance with the Copyright, Designs and Patents Act 1988.

A CIP catalogue record for this book is available from the British Library.

ISBN	978-0-9750472-0-4
DESIGN:	Nikki Dupin
EDITOR:	Zelda Turner
INDEXER:	Caroline Pretty

Printed and bound in Great Britain by Splash Printing Ltd, London

APPI Health Group Ltd, The Chapel, Wellington Rd, NW10 5LJ

www.appihealthgroup.com

WARNING

If you have any medical condition, are pregnant or suffer from back problems, the exercises described in this book should not be followed without first consulting your doctor or seeking expert advice. All guidelines and warnings should be read carefully and the author and publishers cannot accept responsibility for injuries or damage arising out of failure to do so.

WITH THANKS TO: Malin Christenson and Laurent Liotardo for the wonderful photography; to Zelda Turner, Kuo Kang Chen and Nikki Dupin for help with words, pictures and design; and to Elisa's dad, Stephen Stanko, for reading the first draft and encouraging us to continue.

Contents

introduction

Welcome to our new book. We are delighted to have the opportunity to share the APPI Pilates method with you in this way and look forward to the great results that we know you will achieve.

Glenn and I arrived at the APPI method from very different points. And the story of how we got here explains, we think, how our Pilates programme has evolved to be so uniquely accessible to everyone, regardless of experience, fitness level or lifestyle.

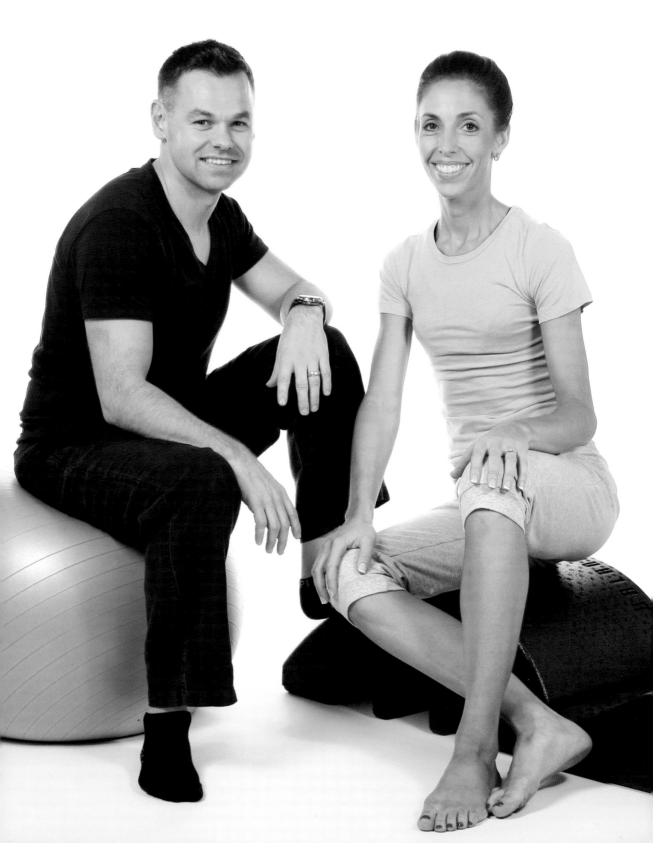

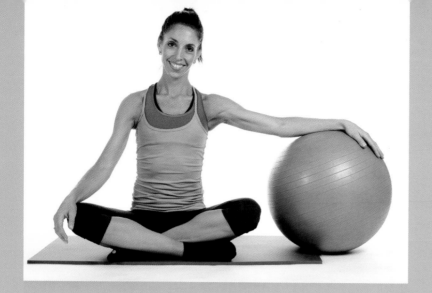
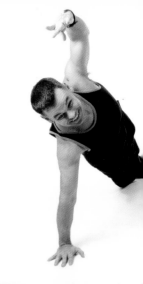

I first started Pilates as a teenager back in Melbourne, Australia. Training as a classical ballerina, I remember our teachers praising the exercises for the way they created long, lean muscles, which allowed greater flexibility and freedom of movement. Pilates honed your body into the ideal form for a ballerina. At the same time, we were told to avoid the gym, running and cycling for fear of bulking up our muscles and/or injuring ourselves.

I loved ballet, but deep down I knew I wasn't going to make it my career. So, at the age of 18, I put my *pointe* shoes away and turned to academia. I had a keen interest in the human body, how it moved and functioned, and its capacity for recovery. So I made up my mind to study Physiotherapy at LaTrobe University in Melbourne. I wanted to learn how to help people recover from injury – and if this could be dance-related, then so much the better.

Taking elective placements in Dance Medicine and Pilates centres, I saw, from the start, that there was a real need for a user-friendly rehabilitation method to help the injured relearn correct and functional movement, together with good posture and muscle balance. Glenn soon shared my vision. Specialising in the elite Sports Medicine centres in the city, he saw how Pilates could become part of athletes' training regimes, helping ensure that the smaller, deep stability muscles become as efficient as the strong powerful outer abdominal and pelvic muscles (a balance that is crucial for preventing injuries).

INTRODUCTION

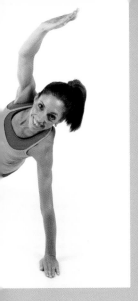
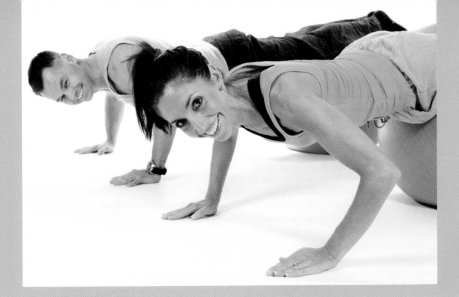

Glenn also experienced first-hand the benefits of Pilates. As a teenager, he had excelled at basketball, and played in the state league in Australia. But shortly after I met him at La Trobe, he sustained a severe back injury that ruled him out of action for a few months. Best to let him tell this part of the story:

'Getting injured was incredibly frustrating, as you can imagine, but Elisa's faith in Pilates proved a crucial turning point for me and my health; I became fascinated by these strange, ballerina-like movements that I was struggling to master, but that were making me better, stronger, more flexible and more agile on the court than I had been for some time. I was struck by how much potential Pilates had in the clinical arena, but when I looked into its use, I realised there was very little to no evidence behind the practice.

'Elisa and I decided that we should look at providing this evidence ourselves. And so, after graduating, a joint scholarship funded our trip to Europe, where we gained insight into the wide variety of traditional and fitness-based Pilates training.

'The more I saw, the more convinced I became that this was an amazing form of exercise. I learnt how to cue movement, how to use visual imagery, how to dissociate my body and move more efficiently. However, I also realised that my patients would struggle with many of the original Pilates movements.

'The length of the leg (the lever) was too long and would hurt someone's back, the starting levels were so high that they would cause pressure on the discs of the lower back, and the analysis of the muscle function was incomplete, in relation to pain and dysfunction.

'Elisa and I decided to review and revise each and every Pilates movement, making them safer and more clinically effective for today's lifestyles, as well as customising them for people with specific injuries. We analysed the exercises on three things: pain, pathology and function, incorporating cutting-edge research on lumbar instability, muscle imbalance and adverse neural tension to develop a modified Pilates programme which would be applicable to people from all walks of life.'

To pick up the story from Glenn: around this time we started working as physiotherapists in the NHS in England, which gave us ample opportunities to apply our method and revise it as required. We realised that there was a real lack of knowledge in the field, in terms of teaching exercise and movement and so, at the request of our colleagues, we started providing informal training courses for any interested physiotherapists.

Over time, these courses became formal, and more numerous, and our method proved highly popular throughout the UK. And then, in 2002, we launched our first Pilates Art Physiotherapy clinic in Hampstead, north London. We had established a reputation among the medical establishment for producing life-changing outcomes for our patients, so clients were referred to us with all sorts of injuries and rehabilitation needs. But from day one, we were also surprised (and delighted!) by the number of people interested in Pilates for reasons of general health and fitness.

Today, we welcome a huge range of people to our clinics, from a child with delayed physical developmental issues to a patient recovering from spinal surgery to an 80-year-old woman wanting to do Pilates to keep active.

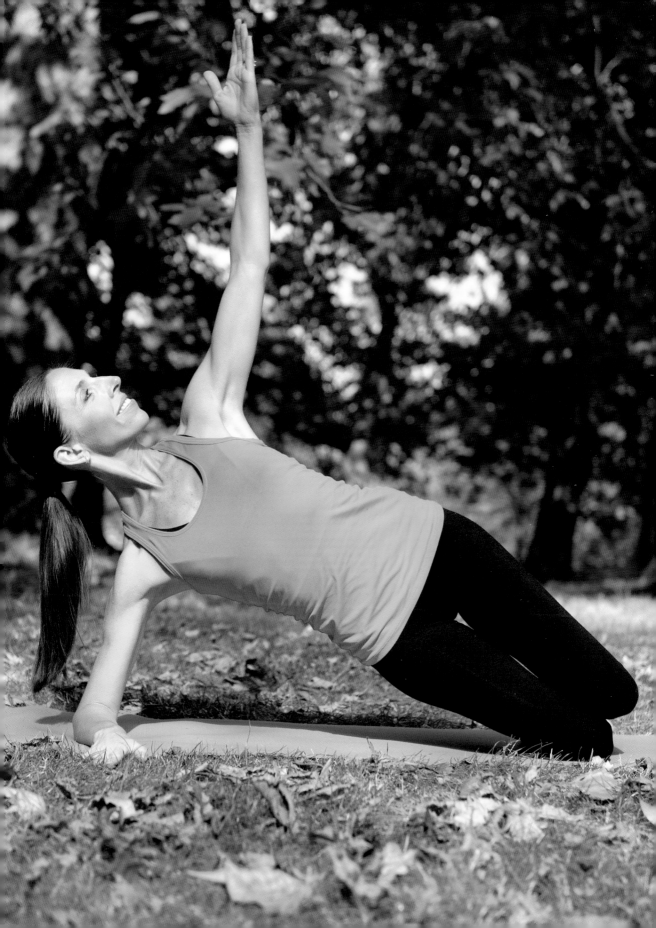

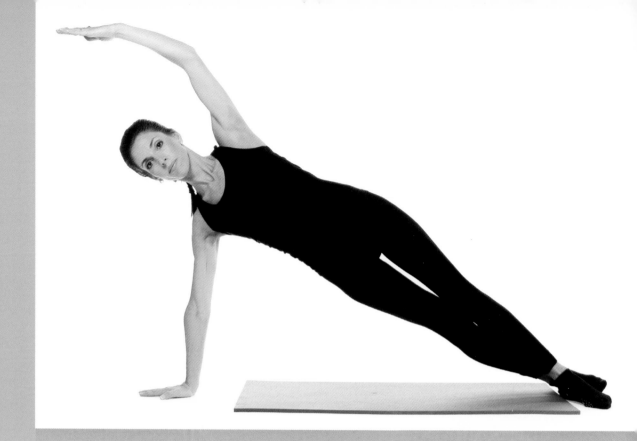

We have APPI centres all over London and within the English National Ballet and Premier League football clubs. APPI-trained physiotherapists work alongside a diverse range of sports stars and performing artists, from the Cirque du Soleil to the UK Olympic team. We deliver modified Pilates programmes across the NHS, the Armed Services, and the UK's police centres. And we now teach a curriculum of 20 different Pilates-based courses in 12 different countries.

Things have changed in my personal life too: these days Glenn and I have two young children and a fast-growing business, so time for myself in the Pilates studio is absolute bliss. For me, regular Pilates practice reminds my body to sit and stand properly and trains my muscles to better hold these good postures.

Despite having done Pilates for many years, my hyper-mobile body needs keeping in check with regular training. Thankfully, my body 'remembers

12   INTRODUCTION

Pilates', so that even if I have missed a few sessions due to the hectic pace of life, it responds to the movements again very quickly. (I promise, yours will too once you've invested a couple of months in this programme.)

I love the way that Pilates tones my body while maintaining flexibility and mobility. There is something far more satisfying for me about practising Pilates compared to working out at the gym, as I know that I am working my body in total control, harmony and balance – just as we were designed to do!

Glenn and I have written this book because we want to motivate you – regardless of your age, fitness level or injury state – to try Pilates. A major driving force behind what we do is our genuine belief in the Pilates method. Ours is a very simple, logical and well-founded approach to teaching people's bodies how to move well in a balanced way. I often say to people that it is not rocket science! It is simply a methodical way of looking at how the body is designed to function and move, enabling you to regain good movement patterns.

The programme is designed to take around six weeks, but it might take you longer to get the hang of these exercises – the important thing is not to rush! If you take your time to focus fully on your own body and movement, your mind and body will totally reap the rewards. Enjoy every minute of focusing on and improving you.

Good luck and enjoy!

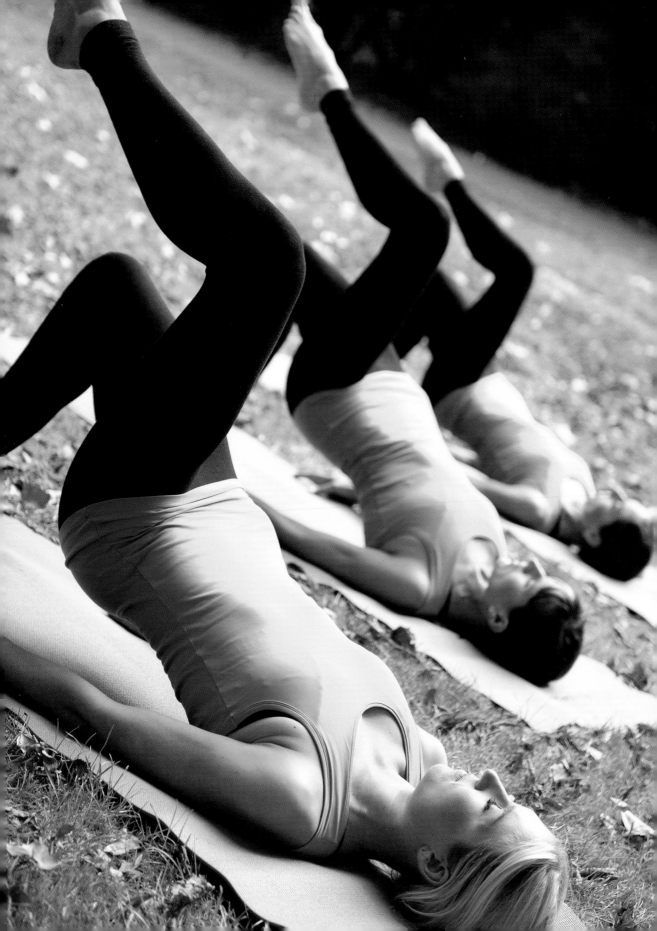

a different kind of workout

'The first requisite to happiness ... is the attainment and maintenance of a uniformly developed body with a sound mind fully capable of naturally, easily and satisfactorily performing our many and varied daily tasks with spontaneous zest and pleasure.'

Joseph Pilates, *Return to Life Through Contrology*

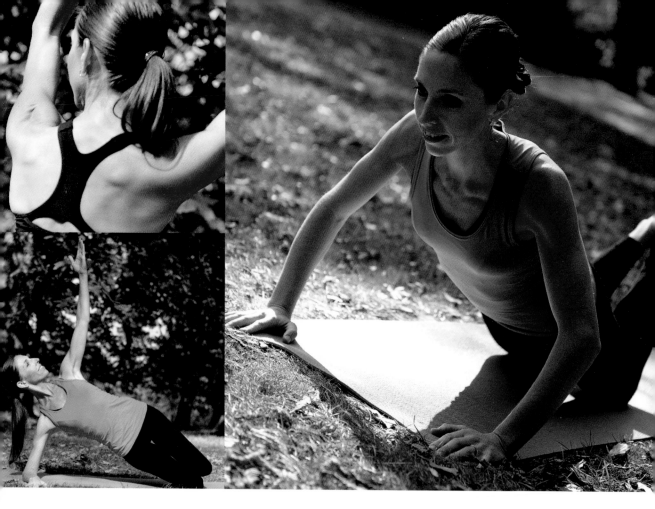

A Different Kind of Workout

The unique method of body-conditioning known as Pilates was invented nearly 100 years ago in Germany by Joseph H. Pilates. Plagued by his own physical shortcomings, caused by a host of childhood ailments, Pilates explored various practices, including yoga, gymnastics, bodybuilding, meditation, and rigorous ancient Greek and Roman regimes, before developing his own exercise technique.

Pilates' genius was to realise that if one system of your body fails, you must develop and strengthen other systems to compensate, in order to restore overall body balance. He refined his exercises whilst interned in an English prisoner of war camp during the First World War and then later, in the 1920s, he opened a studio in New York where his teachings became popular among the dance community.

Pilates' original method was based on 34 movements – published in his 1945 book *Return to Life*. These consisted of strength, mobility and stretching exercises, and were designed to create core stability by engaging the deep abdominal muscles. They were created as a pathway to total health, rather than simply as an exercise regime, for Pilates saw that mental and physical health are interrelated. Thus, if you train the mind to focus entirely on what you wish to achieve, the body can master the precise nature of any movement you ask it to perform.

A New Kind of Pilates

Over the past ten years, we have rigorously reviewed and revised each of Joseph Pilates' 34 mat based movements. A number of these are really only for the supremely flexible, strong and super-fit. Also, Pilates taught his technique, rather like a recipe, in exactly the same way and following the same order for everyone, regardless of ability, posture or injuries.

Our goal has been to make Pilates more adaptable and fit for a vast range of abilities, posture types, ages and personal aims. We believe that Pilates should be available to everyone – whether you are recovering from an injury or simply want to improve your body posture and alignment. So, making use of the latest research, we have created movements that are safer, achievable, and more in line with the way our bodies are designed to function.

The APPI method follows the principles of 'motor relearning', which is the breaking down of whole movements into smaller parts. Once each smaller part is practised and mastered, the elements are put together to recreate the whole movement in a more efficient and natural manner.

The first step in this process is learning how to effectively align the body before activating the deep core of support muscles. Once the deep 'core' has been trained in static and dynamic postures and movements, we then adjust the aim and intensity of each exercise through the use of differing levers (various arm and leg movements), positions (from lying to sitting to standing), and resistance (the use of various small props). And, as you'll find throughout this book, we insist that you take the exercises at your own pace.

What Will Pilates Do For Me?

High-profile fans like Madonna, David Beckham and Nicole Kidman have done much to popularise Pilates, but it has become the fastest-growing exercise technique worldwide for good reasons. Aside from being a more mindful and intelligent exercise approach, it reduces stress and fatigue, and improves alignment and movement control. Unlike gym-based workouts, which can lead to shorter, tighter, bulkier muscles, it will also help to give you lengthened, elongated muscles and promote a more streamlined, balanced body.

Drawing on our background in physiotherapy, the APPI Pilates programme addresses the issue of injuries, fatigue and daily aches through increased body awareness. As Joseph Pilates wrote in *Return to Life*, '[In Pilates] you first purposely acquire complete control of your own body and then through repetition of its exercises, you gradually and progressively acquire that natural rhythm and coordination associated with all your subconscious activities.'

In the early stages of our Pilates programmes, we often observe clients develop good movement control on the mat, before wrestling their way up from the training area, shuffling across the studio, hunching over the water machine and slouching to put their shoes on. Clearly this is not in keeping with the APPI method! Our aim then is to train you to understand your body's posture, balance, capabilities, limitations and normal movement strategies. Throughout this book, you will learn exercises on the mat, but we also teach you how to sit, stand, walk and function better throughout your day, with our Back to Life tips.

As you progress through the programme, you will learn strategies to prevent poor posture and pains creeping back into normal life. Our focus is always on helping you develop a body that is more efficient in daily activities and less prone to future injuries. Establishing strong foundations and a sound understanding of the key elements is crucial and, as with any exercise therapy or new skill, repetition will lead to greater benefits and ability.

As a Pilates beginner, you may feel that there is a lot to think about, worry that the exercises feel too gentle or simply doubt whether you are 'doing it right'. These are all common concerns and the important thing is, don't panic! Instead, reassure yourself that Pilates is a precise method, which targets specific muscles while the body is accurately aligned.

And please remember to view your new Pilates regime as a lifestyle opportunity and not simply as an exercise programme. It will make all the difference!

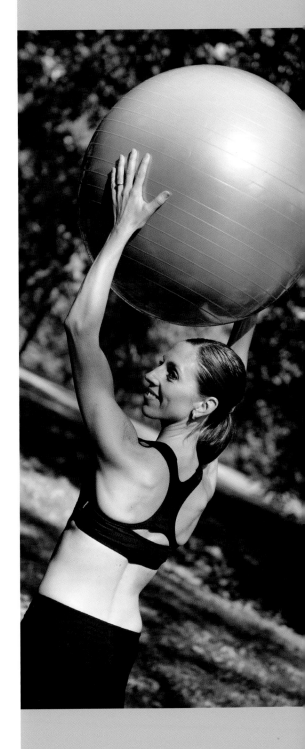

Get to Know Your Body

In order to engage the mind and body harmoniously as one, it will help to understand a little about how your muscular systems function. In Pilates, we talk a lot about your 'centre', by which we mean the local muscle system, consisting of the small, deep, inner layers of muscle and their connective tissue, whose primary role is joint stabilisation.

1. the local muscle system

These local muscles are required to work all day to provide continuous support, and are therefore designed to work at a lower and more gentle rate to avoid fatigue. Along with their deep location, this makes your 'centre' initially difficult to feel in action. A good way to conceptualise the key muscles which make up the local muscular system is to imagine a cylinder of stability located deep within your abdomen.

2. the global muscle system

The global system consists of the larger, outer layers of muscles that generally do not attach directly to joints and whose primary roles are movement and force generation.

A DIFFERENT KIND OF WORKOUT

The Local Muscle System

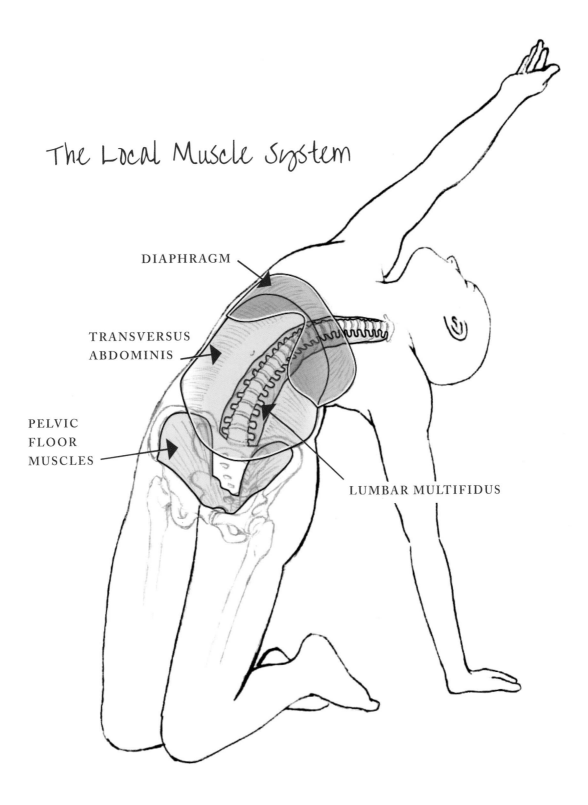

DIAPHRAGM

TRANSVERSUS
ABDOMINIS

PELVIC
FLOOR
MUSCLES

LUMBAR MULTIFIDUS

The primary roles of the global system are the production of movement, force generation and assisting the local muscles in stabilisation when the body's stability is significantly challenged.

A simple way to understand and feel your global muscular system at work is to perform ten sit-ups. In this exercise, your large and powerful rectus abdominis (the most superficial abdominal muscle) is producing the movement. This muscle forms part of the larger and stronger global muscular system, which moves the spine and has no role in direct stabilisation of the individual vertebrae in your back. This is understandable as it does not attach directly to your back and therefore cannot impart direct support.

Within a healthy body, the local and global muscle systems work harmoniously together to meet the changing demands placed on spinal posture and control. The deep local system hums gently away in the background at all times, while the global system enters and departs according to movement, heavy actions required and large challenges to balance and overall orientation. In situations where the body's stability is significantly challenged, the local system acts to stabilise each of the vertebrae in the spine while the global system acts to control the overall orientation of the spine.

It might help to think of the body as an apple. The core of your apple represents the local muscular system – your centre – which is located deep and is crucial to its structure and function. The outer fleshy substance of the apple represents the global muscular system. While you can see and feel the outer global system of the apple, just like you can see and feel the outer and bigger muscles of your global muscular system, you cannot examine the core of the

The Global Muscle System

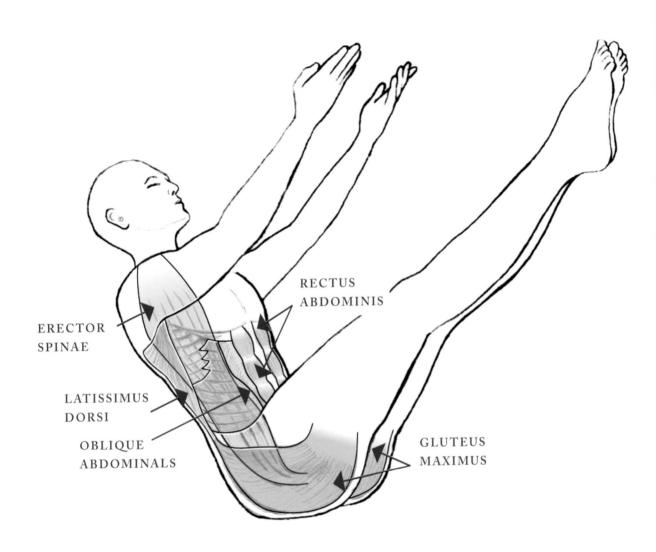

ERECTOR
SPINAE

RECTUS
ABDOMINIS

LATISSIMUS
DORSI

OBLIQUE
ABDOMINALS

GLUTEUS
MAXIMUS

Your deep core or local muscular system,
while being hidden from the outside,
is essential for development and control
of your body.

apple by just looking at it from the outside. Despite this, the apple core is essential to the development and life of the apple itself.

Another way to conceptualise the two muscular systems is to consider the differing body types of a 100m sprinter and a marathon runner. One is stocky, powerful and very bulked up with prominent muscles. This is just like your global system, which works very hard over a short period and exerts a lot of power. Now think of your marathon runner, a much smaller athlete perhaps, yet able to apply constant activity over a longer time. This is your local muscular system, slow acting but providing long-lasting, low-level activity.

When injury occurs, these normal muscle functions go awry. Regardless of the type or cause of injury, the local muscular system is switched off in response to the pain associated with that injury. In contrast, the bigger and more powerful global muscles often spasm or work harder to compensate for the lack of support from your 'centre'. Importantly, the deep, local muscles stay turned off even after the pain has gone and function has returned.

This leaves the vertebrae in the back without ongoing support or protection from a repeat injury. As a consequence, 80 per cent of those suffering back pain will have a recurrence of their pain.

Throughout this book, we will show you how to significantly reduce the likelihood of this recurrence happening through accurate and precise training of the deep muscle centre.

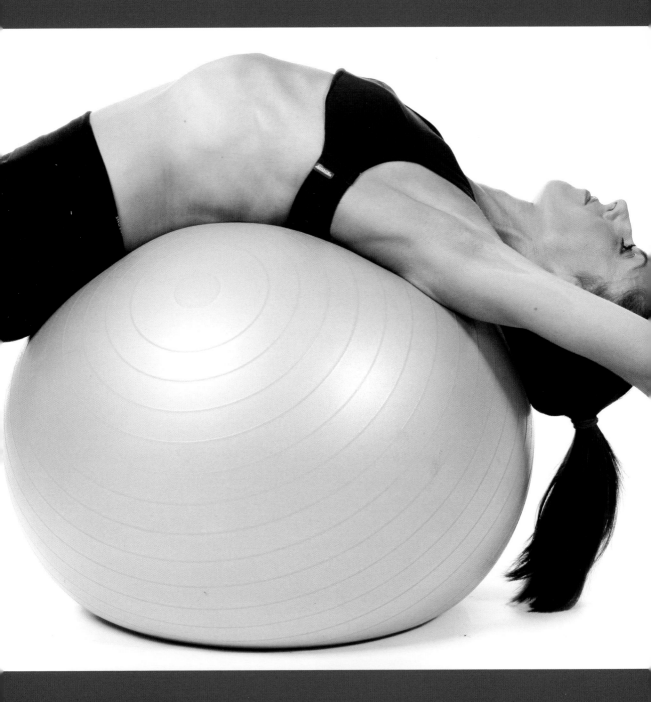

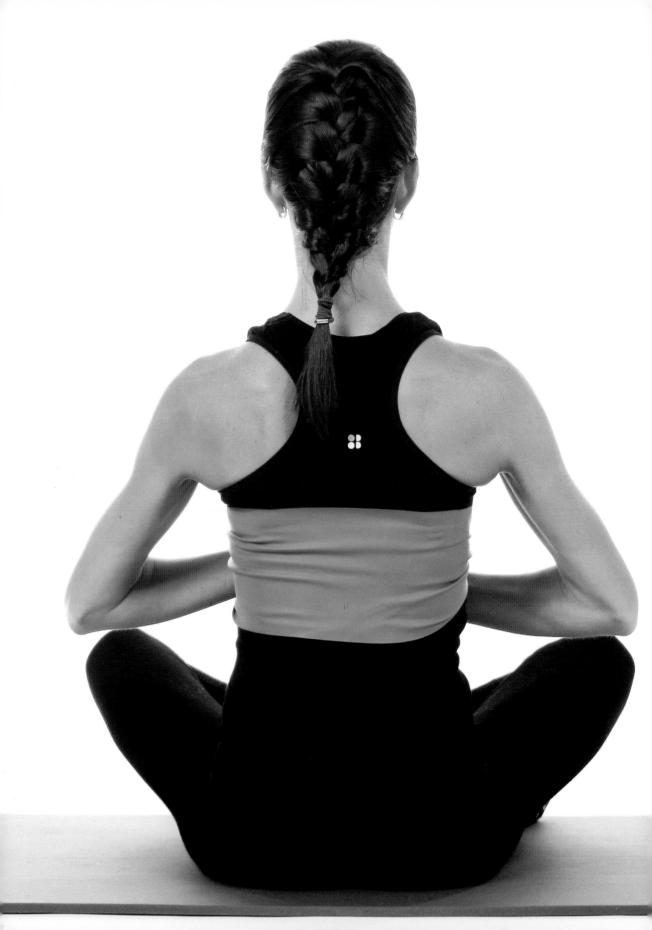

before
you start

Pilates focuses on **eight basic principles**
of general care. Get these right and they
will infuse each exercise with intention
and fullness of expression, as well as
enabling you to incorporate Pilates
into your everyday life.

the *eight* basic principles

1. Concentration

Pilates is about the mind just as much as the body so bring full attention to your starting position and the execution of each movement – don't let yourself get distracted! A common misconception by those with no Pilates experience is that the movements are low level, easy and slow. In fact, Pilates requires absolute, focused commitment in order to get maximum value out of each exercise.

2. Breathing

As Joseph Pilates wrote, 'Breathing is the first act of life, and the last . . . above all, learn how to breathe correctly.' For beginners, learning to breathe properly, inhaling deeply to clear out the lungs of stagnant air, is one of the hardest principles to master. Get it right and it will calm the mind and body, give you better focus and flow of movement, ease muscle tension and even help mobilise the joints.

3. Centring

Pilates always starts by bringing the focus to the centre or core of your body – what Joseph Pilates termed your 'Powerhouse'. APPI Pilates is uniquely founded on highly precise and accurate centring, no matter what level of Pilates experience or body type you have. Over the next six weeks (and beyond), we will work to ensure successful 'centring' and then progressively challenge control of the centre through various arm and leg movements, positions and props.

4. Control

Every Pilates exercise is done with accuracy and complete muscular control. No body part is left to its own devices. Learn control, and you are on your way to mastering the art of efficient movement in everyday life.

BEFORE YOU START

5. Precision

Precision is about performing the exercise correctly. Mindful focus during and after a Pilates movement, along with routine practice, will lead to precision – as the old saying goes, 'Practice does not make perfect. Only perfect practice makes perfect'.

6. Flowing Movements

Once a movement is started in Pilates, you flow through the motions until the number of repetitions is reached or you feel you are losing control of your centre. If you observe people who are experienced in Pilates, you will notice their effortless and continuous flow of movement – everything appears seamless, with no sense of a 'start' or a 'finish'.

7. Integrated Isolation

Pilates recognises the body as a finely tuned, harmonious system, where complete muscle integration creates precise and flowing movements. Once the art of centring is accomplished, APPI Pilates teaches you how to maintain your core abdomino-pelvic support while performing isolated movements of the body, leading to the ability to maintain the same support in everyday functional positions (sitting, standing, etc), while executing complex, daily movements such as typing at the computer or pushing a pram.

8. Routine

APPI Pilates is based on a motor relearning programme, and routine is vital to its success. To fully gain the benefits you must do at least 30 minutes of Pilates every day, and ensure that you can complete your session from start to finish without interruptions.

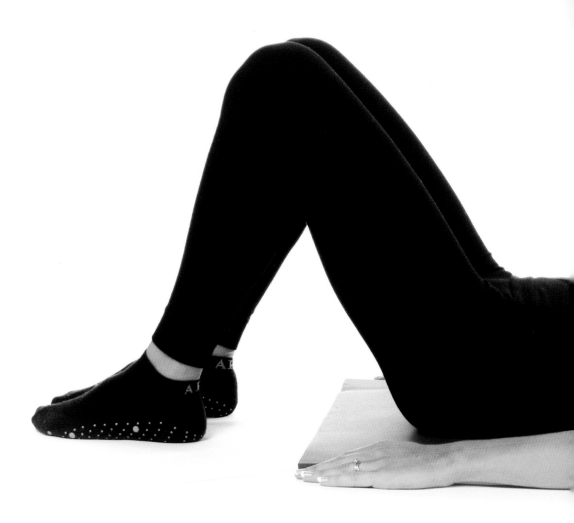

The Pilates rest position

Learning the rest position is the first step to beginning your Pilates programme.

Lie on your back in the centre of the mat. If you feel that your chin is poking upwards, place a small head cushion or folded towel under the base of your head. Bend your knees to right angles and place your feet on the floor, hip distance apart, directly in line with your sitting bones (the bony prominences deep in your buttocks).

BEFORE YOU START

To release unwanted tension around your lower back, imagine your pelvis as a heavy anchor sinking slowly down through the floor.

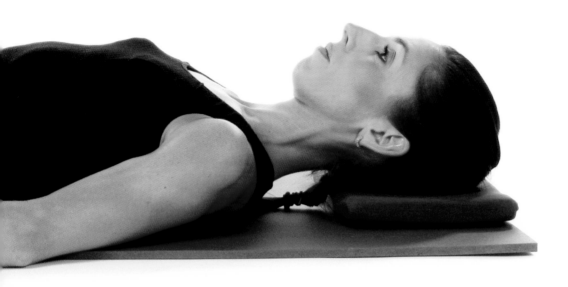

To relax the muscles in your upper back, allow the back of your ribcage to rest into the mat. To help with this, imagine the back of your ribcage making a broad impression in the mat underneath you. Take a breath in to the very sides and back of your ribcage and imagine this impression broadening and deepening. Place your arms down long beside you on the mat. To open the front of your chest and guide your shoulder blades onto your ribcage, imagine your collarbones gently widening.

Your body is now aligned in the Pilates rest position. This position should feel relaxed and not forced.

the five key elements

The Five Key Elements are the essential building blocks of the technique. Learn them in the Pilates rest position *(see over)* for ease of movement.

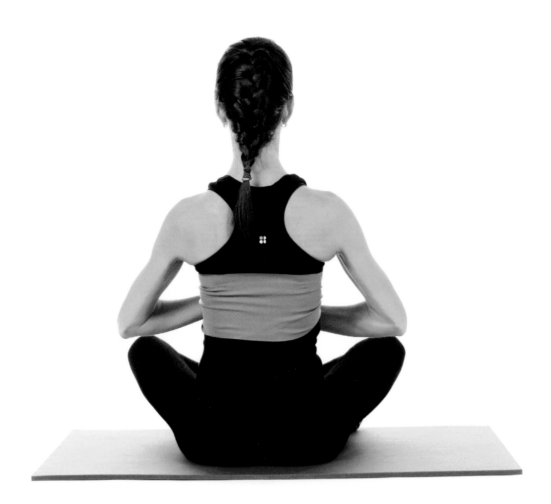

1. lateral breathing

Aim to breathe in wide and full into the sides and back of your ribcage.

When inhaling correctly, you will notice that the lower half of the ribcage expands widthways as well as becoming deeper from front to back. When exhaling, aim to relax all the muscles of the ribcage completely. Remember that exhalation is a passive function consisting largely of passive elastic recoil and relaxation. Breathing correctly promotes the efficient exchange of gases and avoids a build-up of any unnecessary muscular tension.

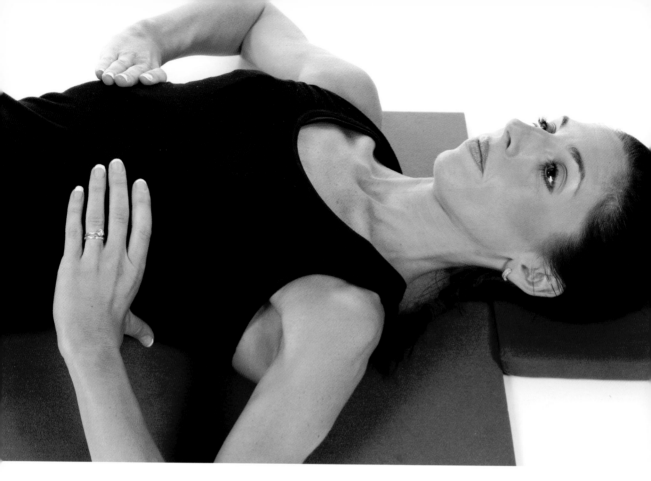

• *Breathing exercise one*

Increase awareness of your natural breath patterns.

Assume the Pilates rest position. Without trying to alter the way you normally breathe, take a few breaths in and out. Pay attention to where your breath is going. Ask yourself the following questions:

➤ Where do you feel movement occurring?
➤ Do you feel movement of your ribcage, stomach or shoulders?
➤ If you feel your ribcage moving, is it moving width-wise, poking upwards or arching as you breathe in?
➤ How full is your breath?
➤ Do you feel any tension as you breathe out?

BEFORE YOU START

- ## *Breathing exercise two*
  Learn lateral breathing in a comfortable rest position.

Assume the Pilates rest position and place your hands on the lower half of your ribcage.

Take a breath in and imagine the lower half of your ribcage becoming wider and deeper. It can help to think of breathing the lower half of your ribcage deeper into the mat underneath you. Keep your upper chest, neck and shoulders relaxed. Exhale and imagine the sides of your lower ribcage sinking towards one another. Repeat this deeper and wider breath pattern a few times. Notice how your fingertips draw away from one another as you breathe in and then lace towards one another as you breathe out.

- ## *Breathing exercise three*
  Learn lateral breathing mechanics whilst sitting.

Sit upright on a chair with even weight through your sitting bones. Place your feet hip distance apart on the floor. Check that your ribcage is positioned directly over your pelvis and your head is held upright. Take a Pilates band or scarf and wrap this snugly around the lower half of your ribcage. Hold the two ends of your Pilates band in one hand and relax the other hand onto your lap.

Imagine your collarbones widening and your shoulder blades melting downwards. Take a breath in and imagine the lower half of your ribcage becoming wider and deeper. When breathing correctly, you will notice your ribcage expanding into your Pilates band as you breathe in and then drawing away from the Pilates band as you breathe out. Remember to keep your upper chest, neck and shoulders relaxed.

2. centring

Your Pilates 'centre' refers to the deep abdominal cylinder of muscles that provides crucial support to your spine and pelvis.

This cylinder comprises your deepest abdominal muscle, the transversus abdominis, your pelvic floor, diaphragm and multifidus muscles, found deep in your back. A finely tuned and efficient centre of deep abdomino-pelvic muscles is one of the fundamental requirements for a strong and stable spinal posture.

'Centring' refers to engaging these muscles in unison while keeping the lower back in the 'neutral' spine position (ie the natural inwards C curve of the lower back). We are born with four natural spinal curvatures. Look at the body from the side and you will observe two small inward spinal curves at the neck and lower back regions, and two small outwards curves at the upper back and lower pelvic (sacral) areas of the spine.

Depending on your lifestyle choices (athletic or sedentary), these natural curves may be unnaturally exaggerated or reduced. If your body has aligned itself incorrectly, the solution lies in repositioning your lower back into the neutral spine position and engaging your centre before starting any Pilates movement.

'Centring' refers to engaging these muscles in unison while keeping the lower back in the 'neutral' spine position (ie the inwards C curve of the lower back).

BEFORE YOU START

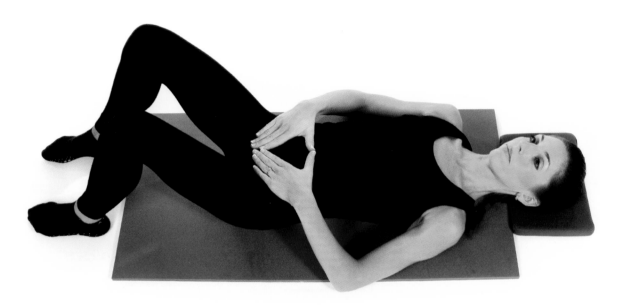

- *Neutral spine position*

  Learn to position your lower back in the neutral spine position.

Assume the Pilates rest position. With your thumbs in your belly button, place your fingertips on your pubic bone and then flatten the heels of your hands wide onto the bony sides of your pelvis. Imagine these four points forming a diamond shape on the front of your pelvis.

Gently roll the bottom point of the diamond towards the floor (creating an arch in your lower back). Now gently roll the top point of the diamond towards the floor (flattening your lower back). Repeat several times. To find your neutral position, rest the pelvic diamond in the middle position of these two movements, where all points of the diamond are level.

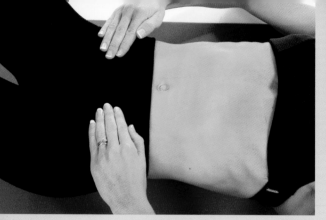
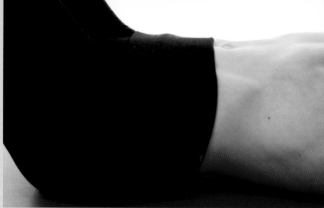

- *Centring exercise one*

  Learn how to engage your centre by activating the deep abdominal muscles.

Assume the Pilates rest position. Place your fingertips onto the bony prominences on the sides of your pelvis. Now, move your fingertips one inch inwards and downwards so that they are placed directly over the deep internal oblique and transversus abdominis muscle, ready to feel your centre engage.

Imagine the deep abdominal muscles as a supportive muscular corset with ten notches far below the belly button, just like a low-slung belt. Take a breath in and then breathe out all the way. Before taking your next breath in, slowly and gently draw in your muscular corset from below the belly button onto the first or second notch only, to engage your deep abdominal muscles. There should be no movement of your back. When setting your centre correctly, the muscles under your fingers should gently and slowly tighten and should not bulge. Hold this gentle abdominal contraction now and keep breathing normally. After a few breaths, slowly release the abdominal contraction while keeping your lower back in its neutral position.

HELP FROM THE PHYSIO

> Slowly and gently draw in your lower tummy. Gently draw your tummy away from the line of your trousers. Imagine your lower tummy drawing towards the front of your spine.

BEFORE YOU START

- ## *Centring exercise two*

   Learn how to set your centre by activating the
   pelvic floor muscles.

Assume the Pilates rest position. Place your fingertips onto the bony prominences on the sides of your pelvis. Now move your fingertips one inch inwards and downwards from these bony prominences. Your fingertips are now placed directly over the deep internal oblique and transversus abdominis muscle ready to feel your centre engage.

Imagine the pelvic floor muscles as a supportive net running from the pubic bone at the front of the pelvis to the tailbone at the back of the pelvis. This net is made up of multiple layers of muscle and supportive tissue. Take a breath in and then breathe all the way out. Before taking your next breath in, slowly and gently draw the pelvic floor net upwards. There should be no movement of your back. When setting your centre correctly, the muscles under your fingers should gently and slowly tighten and should not bulge. Hold this gentle pelvic floor contraction now and keep breathing normally. After a few breaths, slowly release the pelvic floor contraction while keeping your lower back in its neutral position.

Now that you have practised two different methods of setting your Pilates centre, decide which method feels best for you. When setting your centre use either the muscular corset or the pelvic floor cue. Ensure the muscles under your fingers gently and slowly tighten and do not bulge into your fingers. This 'bulge' sensation is the action of your internal oblique abdominal muscles and is probably an indication that you are using too much effort. To activate your Pilates centre in isolation, you should use a very gentle effort and be precise in your muscular focus. This is vital in targeting the specific muscles that support the spine and ultimately in gaining control of lower back pain.

3. ribcage placement

To achieve optimal spinal alignment, the ribcage should be positioned directly over the pelvis when looking at the body from the side in sitting or standing.

When you are lying on your back, the entire back of the ribcage should rest naturally on the mat rather than arching away from the mat. Incorrect alignment can take the form of a forwards 'flaring' or a backwards 'sway' of the ribcage. When lying on the mat, it can help to imagine the ribcage 'sinking into the floor' or 'softening the breastbone' to achieve a more ideal alignment. In sitting or standing, imagine a spring connecting the bottom of the ribcage to the hip bones on either side of the body.

- *Ribcage placement with arm lifts*
  Challenge correct alignment of the ribcage.

Assume the Pilates rest position. Float your arms upwards, bringing your hands over your shoulders with your palms inwards.

Begin by relaxing the back of your ribcage into the mat underneath you. To do this, focus on a few natural breaths in and out. As you breathe in, breathe in wide and deep to the back of your ribcage and feel it expand in the mat underneath you. Engage your centre. Then, lower your arms overhead as far as possible while keeping the back of your ribcage on the mat. Ensure that you do not arch your back or 'flare' your ribcage forwards off the mat. Move your arms forwards to bring your hands over your shoulders again. Repeat this movement up to ten times and pay attention to keeping your ribcage feeling broad across the mat underneath you.

BEFORE YOU START

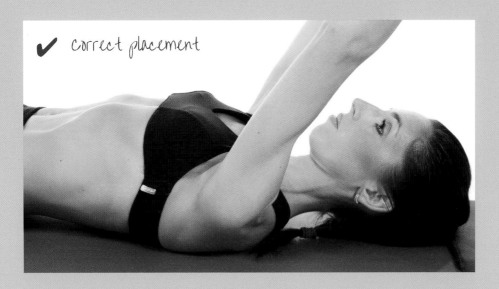

✔ correct placement

You can start developing body awareness in upright postures by practising this exercise in sitting.

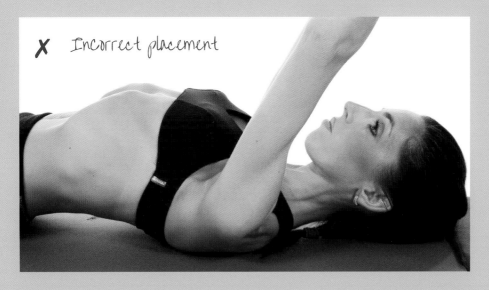

✗ Incorrect placement

4. shoulder blade placement

Poor shoulder blade stability can lead to a plethora of problems, from overuse of the upper shoulder blade and neck muscles to significant neck and shoulder pain.

Whether stability has been compromised by injury or simply by too much slouching, our aim here is to create awareness of the muscles responsible as well as to teach you some techniques for setting the shoulder blades into optimal posture.

- *Shoulder blade setting*

  Counteract the effects of your sedentary lifestyle by setting your shoulder blades correctly on your ribcage throughout the day.

Assume the Pilates rest position. Set your shoulder blades into good posture by slowly and gently widening your collarbones. When performed correctly, you will feel the lower half of your shoulder blades gently draw downwards on to your ribcage. Your neck and upper back muscles remain relaxed and there is no movement of your ribcage or head.

- *Shoulder blade isolations* *(forwards and backwards on the ribcage)*

  Learn body awareness of shoulder blade movement and activate the muscles of the shoulder blade.

Assume the Pilates rest position. Float your arms upwards, bringing your hands over your shoulders with your palms inwards.

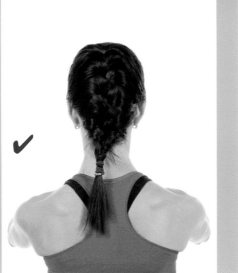 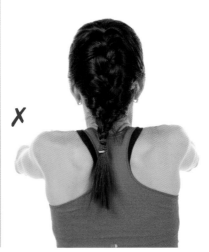

Reach upwards from the base of your shoulder blade, through your arms and fingertips to reach for the ceiling. With the correct movement, you will feel your shoulder blades gently glide upwards from the mat. Keep your head, neck and ribcage still and focus on the movement of your shoulder blades only. Then gently glide your shoulder blades back onto the mat. Keep your arms long throughout the movement and again focus on the movement of the shoulder blade only. Repeat up to ten times and aim for a smooth forwards and backwards gliding movement of your shoulder blades on your ribcage.

- *Shoulder blade isolations* *(upwards and downwards on the ribcage)*
  Learn body awareness of shoulder blade movement and activate the upper and lower fibres of the trapezius muscle of the shoulder blade.

Assume the Pilates rest position. Glide your shoulder blades up towards your ears and then down to the rest position. Your arms should remain resting long beside you on the mat. Ensure that you keep the collarbones feeling wide across the front of your chest. Repeat this movement up to ten times and aim for a smooth upwards and downwards gliding movement of your shoulder blades on your ribcage. Once you have developed awareness of your shoulder blade alignment in the rest position, practise these exercises in sitting.

THE FIVE KEY ELEMENTS

5. head and neck placement

For ideal posture and the prevention of headaches and painful neck conditions, the natural curve of the neck needs to be maintained.

When the body is observed from the side, there is a small natural inward curve in the neck. The neck is held in this natural position by the deep stabilising muscles of the neck, called the deep neck flexors. You can imagine these muscles as broad supportive bands running deeply from the top to the bottom of the front of your neck. Body awareness is the first step to correcting 'forward head' (and slouched upper body) posture in your own body.

- ## *Head and neck posture*
  Learn awareness of correct head and neck posture.

Assume the Pilates rest position. Slowly and gently nod your chin towards your chest – this is a pure nodding movement of your head on the top bone in your neck. Keep the muscles on the front of your neck and jaw relaxed. It may help to place your tongue on the roof of your mouth and keep your jaw slightly apart. Once you have developed body awareness of your head and neck alignment in the rest position, you can practise this exercise sitting. Concentrate on:

- ➤ Lengthening the back of your neck.
- ➤ Imagining a string on the crown of your head gently being drawn to lengthen your neck.
- ➤ Extending the crown of your head away from your tailbone.
- ➤ Imagining your head as a helium balloon floating upwards.

BEFORE YOU START

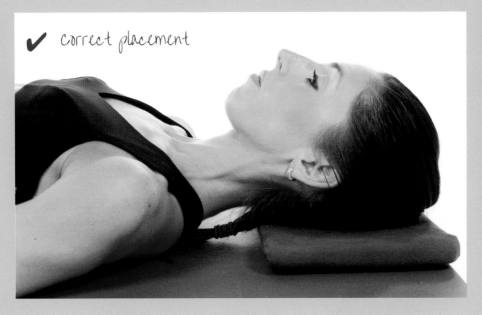

✔ correct placement

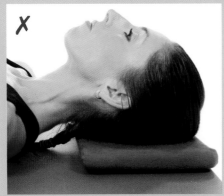

✗

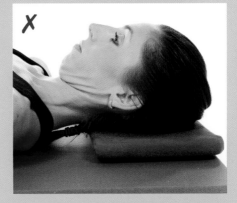

✗

It will take time and practice to adopt the **Five Key Elements**. Persistent practice is key to moving forward with confidence, ease and energy.

watch points

Use these pages for reference, at any point in your Pilates programme, to check that you are avoiding common pitfalls.

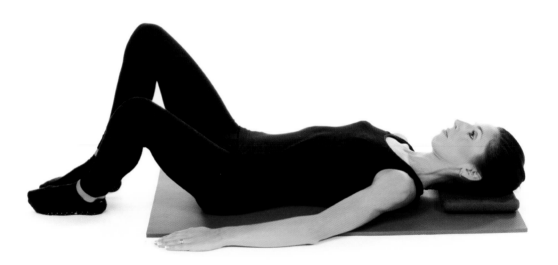

When exercising supine

- Maintain a deep connection with your centre to avoid arching your back.
- Don't overdo it! Remember, Pilates is not the gym – you will not feel the 'burn' with these exercises. Don't force, grip or stop breathing.

- Keep your upper body, shoulders and neck relaxed throughout the exercise.
- Allow your head and neck to sink down into the mat and keep the back of your neck long.
- Avoid any unwanted downwards pressure through your arms or legs.
- Prevent your collarbones from rolling inwards by keeping them wide.
- Maintain even weight through the key points of your feet.
- Keep breathing smoothly and gently into the sides and back of the ribcage. If you are holding your breath, you are probably forcing your muscles too hard. Try again with less effort so that your ribcage can expand naturally.
- Keep your buttocks relaxed throughout the movement.

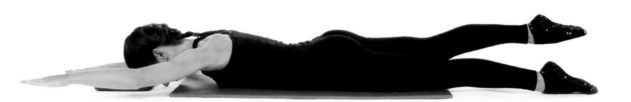

When exercising on your tummy

- Do not let your body sink into the mat. Maintain good centring to avoid flaring your ribcage into the mat.
- To avoid arching your lower back, imagine your tailbone reaching for your heels.
- Avoid downward pressure through your arms.
- Keep your collarbones wide and your shoulder blades gliding downwards.
- Maintain a gentle chin nod to keep the back of your neck long.
- Keep your buttocks relaxed throughout the movement.

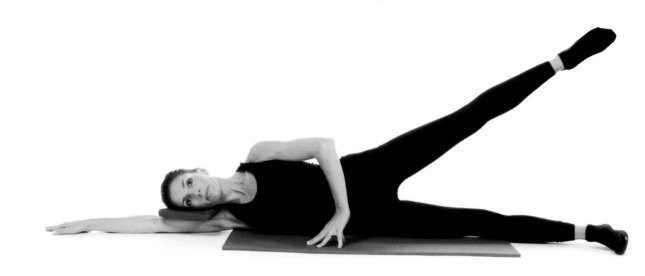

When exercising on your side

- Keep your back and pelvis still – movements should come from your hip joints only.
- Imagine balancing cups of tea on your top shoulder and hip to prevent them rocking during movement.
- Avoid downwards pressure through your top hand and place it onto your hip once you feel in control.
- Ensure that your head and neck remain fully relaxed into your supporting cushion.
- Keep your ribcage soft: gravity acts to flare it forwards in this position.
- Remember to keep the waist lengthened on both sides.

When exercising in four-point kneeling

- Focus on maintaining the deep abdominal connection throughout the movement to avoid arching your lower back. When centring, feel the movement of your abdominal wall drawing inwards towards the front of your spine – don't let it sag towards the mat.

- Keep equally long on both sides of your trunk to avoid hip hitching during leg movements. Keep your arms long but avoid locking the elbow joints.
- Avoid sinking downwards into your shoulder blades and instead think of lifting your breastbone away from the mat.
- If you have any knee discomfort, place a cushion under your knees.
- Maintain a gentle chin nod to stabilise your head and neck – it is key to activating the deep neck muscles, which support your head and neck.

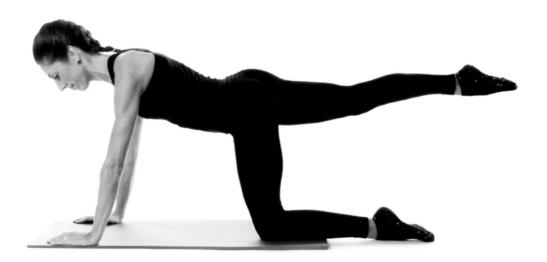

As you progress through the APPI programme – from beginner Pilates to intermediate to advanced – you will notice that some of the exercises are repeated, with increased challenges (for example, our programme takes you from Hundreds: Level 1 to Level 4). As you stretch yourself with the more difficult techniques, remind yourself of the specific watch points detailed in the earlier levels of those movements.

the basic rules . . .

- Read through and understand the exercises you're about to do – taking heed of the **Physio's Help** points.

- Do not skip your **Warm Up** or your **Cool Down** (these exercises make up your training programme in week 1).

- Take time to align your body, as instructed, before commencing each movement. This will help brain and body connect.

- At the end of each week, the **Checklist** will help you decide whether you are ready to progress to the next level.

- Go at your own pace – you do not have to finish the programme within six weeks.

- If at any stage you feel you are not ready to progress or simply wish to consolidate the current exercises, continue practising the programme that you are confident with. Pilates is about quality, not quantity!

- Learn how to incorporate Pilates into your daily life with our weekly **Back to Life** tips.

At no stage should you experience any worsening ache or pain. If you do, stop the exercise and consult your physiotherapist or GP.

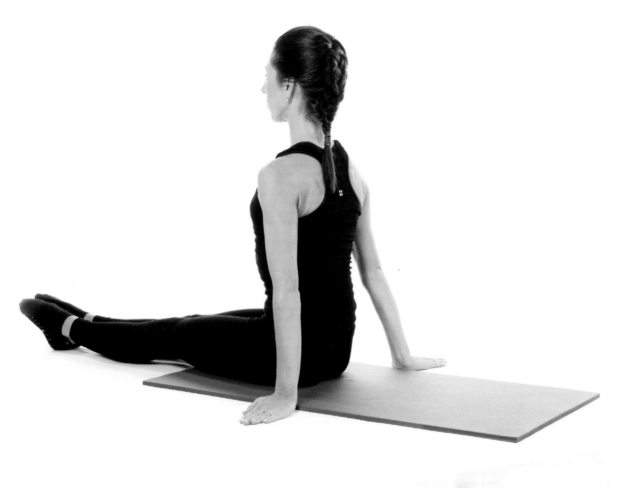

A small number of props will help you get the most out of your Pilates programme. You may think about investing in the following:

- a small or large Pilates head cushion

- a Pilates sitting block

- a Pilates band to help with stretching

- a pair of massage balls to release tight muscles.

WHAT YOU NEED:

✓ **1.** A suitable space for your Pilates session – you should be able to lie fully stretched and have room to move your arms and legs freely around you

✓ **2.** An exercise mat

✓ **3.** A thin (one-inch) cushion or folded towel

✓ **4.** A supportive pillow

✓ **5.** A small ball or extra towel rolled up into a small log

✓ **6.** A scarf (or Pilates stretch band)

✓ **7.** A bottle of water

THE BASIC RULES

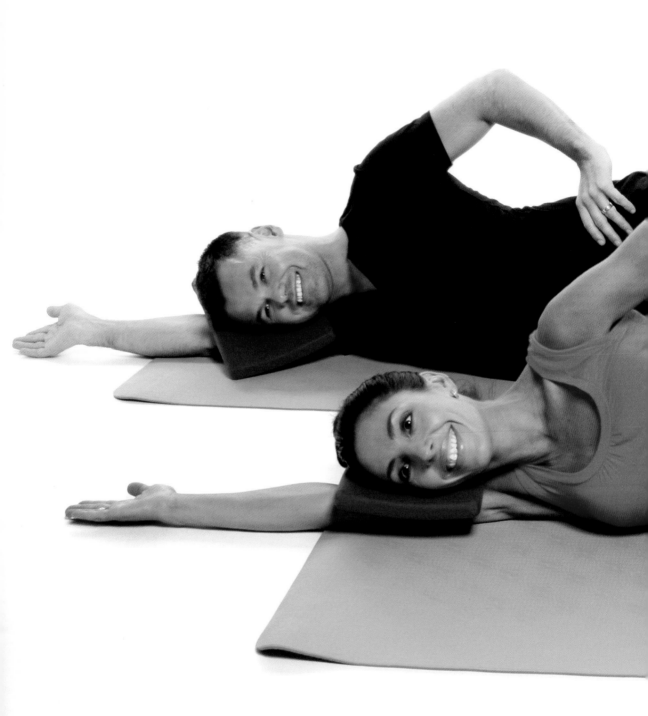

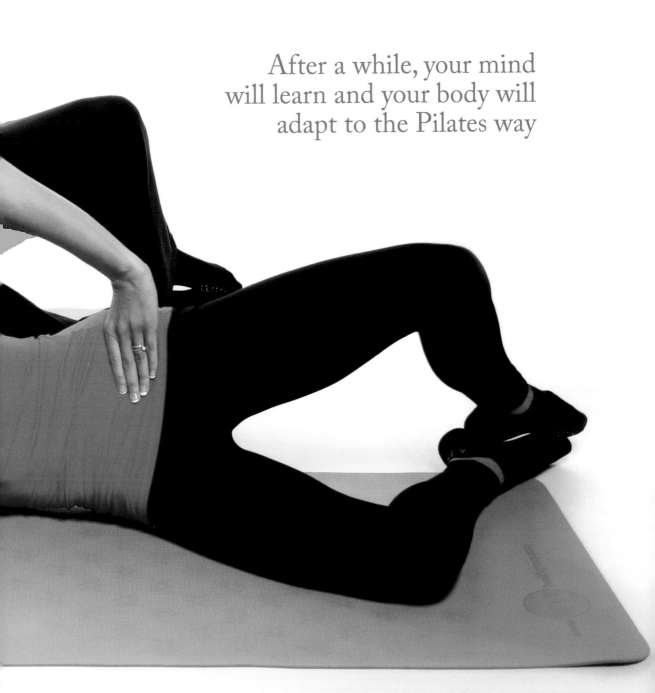

After a while, your mind
will learn and your body will
adapt to the Pilates way

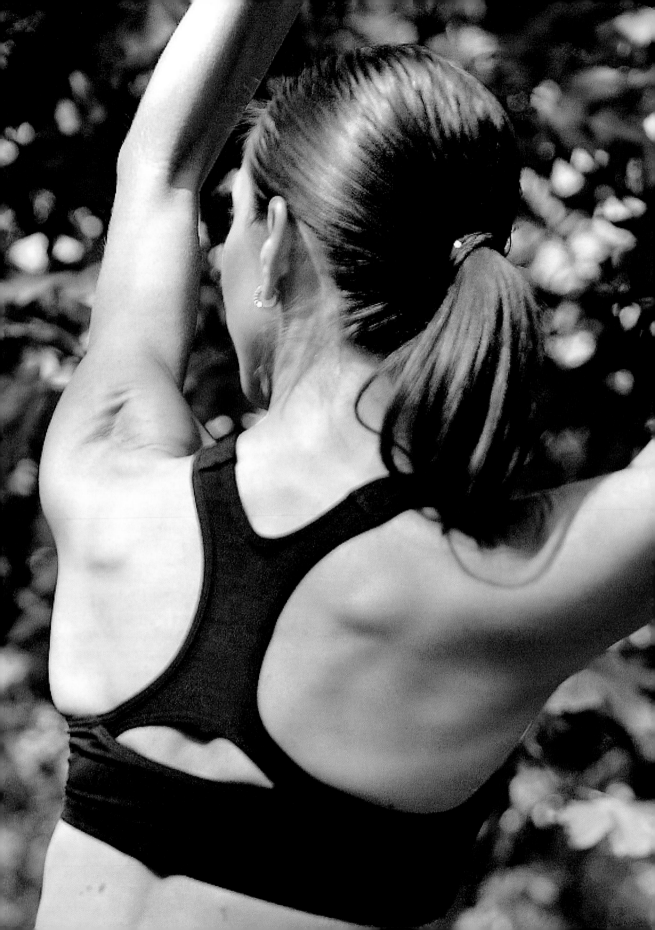

week 1

... is where you learn the basic exercises that will later become part of your daily **Warm Up** and **Cool Down**

1. hundreds *(level one)*

Combines endurance training of the abdominal 'centre' with lateral breathing and accurate body alignment.

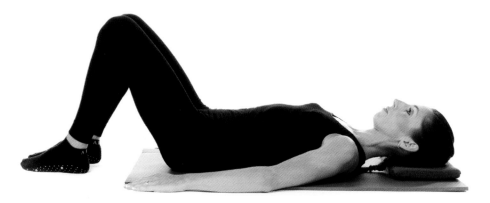

Assume the Pilates rest position. Breathe in to prepare. As you breathe out, slowly and gently draw in your lower abdominal or pelvic floor muscles to engage your centre. Now, breathe normally for up to ten breaths while maintaining the connection with your centre and neutral spine alignment. To finish, slowly release your centre while maintaining neutral spine alignment.

HELP FROM THE PHYSIO

➤ Place your fingertips on the bony points at the front of your pelvis, then move in and down an inch to position on your centring muscles. If you cough, you will feel the muscles under your fingertips bulge rapidly – these are the more superficial abdominal muscles and not your deep centring muscles. Slowly and gently set your centre, aiming to feel a slow drawing in of the muscles under your fingertips.

➤ To aid awareness, place a thin cushion under the small of your back. Relax your back fully onto the cushion to support neutral alignment – remove as your control and awareness improve. Don't squeeze your buttock muscles – it's not necessary!

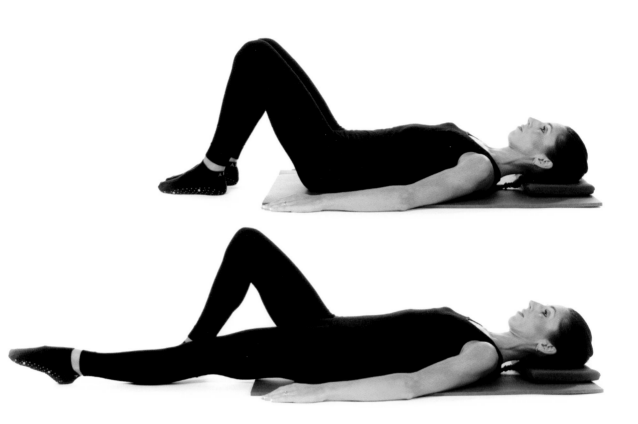

2. one leg stretch *(level one)*

Trains stability of your lower back and pelvis during coordinated movement of your legs.

Lie in the Pilates rest position. Gently engage your centre. Breathe in to prepare. Breathe out as you slide your right heel forwards along the mat to lengthen your leg fully. Breathe in as you slide your heel back in along the floor. Repeat up to 10 times, alternating legs.

HELP FROM THE PHYSIO

➤ Imagine your toe reaching forwards to touch a button on the wall in front of you but do not arch your back.

➤ To mobilise the nerves, which run from your spine down the back of your leg, lead with your heel as you lengthen your leg away. Imagine that your heel is now reaching for that button. Reach with your leg and not your pelvis.

➤ To prevent your pelvis from rocking sideways, imagine that it is anchored in a block of cement.

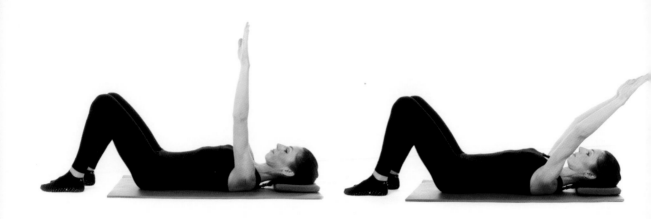

3. double leg stretch *(level one)*

Trains awareness and stability of your back during coordinated arm (and in later levels, leg) movements.

Lie in the Pilates rest position. Gently engage your centre. Lift your arms to shoulder height, keeping them long and your palms facing outwards.

Breathe in to prepare. Breathe out and lower your arms overhead, keeping your ribcage still and the back of your neck long. As you breathe in, draw an outwards circle with each arm, finishing the movement with your hands lifted above your shoulders again. Repeat up to ten circles in one direction and then up to ten circles in the opposite direction. Breathe out and lower your arms to the mat.

HELP FROM THE PHYSIO

➤ Avoid arching your back or ribcage. Throughout the movement, imagine the soft imprint of your ribcage on the mat underneath you.

➤ If you feel any neck tension, relax by lengthening the back of your neck, opening your jaw slightly and placing your tongue on the roof of your mouth.

➤ Keep your hands at least shoulder-width apart so that your collarbones and chest remain wide and open.

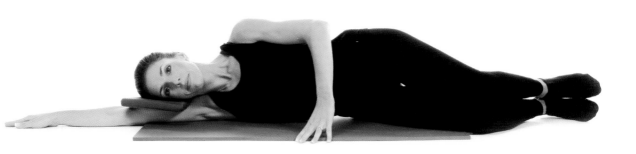

4. the clam *(level one)*

Isolates and strengthens the deep stabilising gluteal muscles of your hip and pelvis.

Lie on one side with your hips and shoulders stacked, your knees bent and your thighs just forwards of your body. Find the neutral position of your pelvis and lengthen your waist equally on both sides. Keep your lower arm extended under your head and your top hand on the mat for light support. Place a small cushion under your head. Gently engage your centre.

Breathe in to prepare. Breathe out as you lift your top knee upwards, keeping your feet together and your pelvis and waist still. Breathe in as you lower your top leg. Repeat up to 10 times on each leg.

HELP FROM THE PHYSIO

> If you are still struggling to feel the right muscles, move your top hand forwards on the mat and roll your body forwards to work against gravity more.

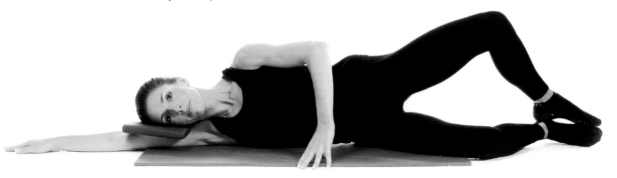

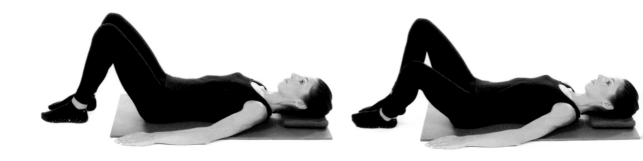

5. hip twist *(level one)*

Challenges your ability to move your hips while maintaining stability of your back and pelvis, enabling efficient movement in everyday activities such as walking and climbing stairs.

Lie in the Pilates rest position. Gently engage your centre. Breathe in to prepare. Breathe out as you move one knee outwards, maintaining the neutral spine position. Keep your foot on the mat and allow it to roll onto its outer side. Breathe in and move your knee inwards in line with your hip and place your foot flat on the mat. Repeat up to 10 times, alternating legs.

HELP FROM THE PHYSIO

➤ Avoid arching your back or ribcage. Throughout the movement, imagine the soft imprint of your ribcage on the mat underneath you.

➤ If you feel any neck tension, relax by lengthening the back of your neck, opening your jaw slightly and placing your tongue on the roof of your mouth.

➤ Keep your hands at least shoulder-width apart so that your collarbones and chest remain wide and open.

➤ Prevent your shoulder blades from hitching upwards by imaging a small helium balloon cushioning the space between your ears and your shoulders.

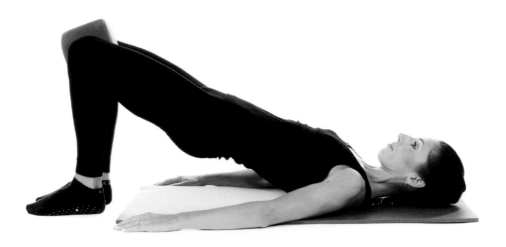

6. shoulder bridge *(level one)*

Mobilise your back while strengthening key muscles to improve pelvic stability.

Lie in the Pilates rest position. To avoid any unwanted pressure through your neck, remove any pillows from under your head. Gently engage your centre. Breathe in to prepare. As you breathe out, gently roll your lower back into the mat, float your tailbone up off the mat and continue to peel your spine away from the mat, until you are resting on your shoulder blades. Breathe in and hold the shoulder bridge position. As you breathe out, roll back down through your back one bone at a time until you resume the neutral spine starting position. Repeat up to 10 times.

HELP FROM THE PHYSIO

➤ Keep your movement slow and aim to peel away one bone at a time. You have seventeen bones in your upper and lower back alone, so don't rush this. Instead, imagine your spine as a chain and aim to lift one link away at a time.

➤ Avoid hyper-extending your lower back by checking that your hips are higher than your ribcage and focus on lengthening your lower back.

➤ If you feel cramping at the back of your thighs, your hamstring muscles are overworking and your glutes underworking. Imagine drawing your sitting bones together as you roll your pelvis off the mat to engage the gluteal muscles. Do not roll onto your neck.

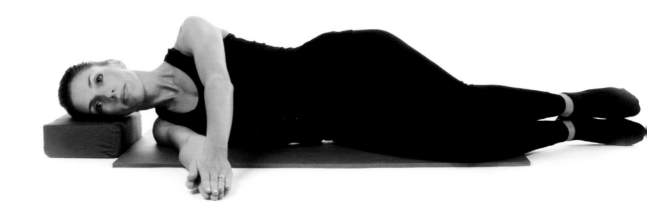

7. arm openings

Promotes mobility of your upper back while opening and stretching the front of your chest.

Lie on one side with your head on a cushion, your shoulders and hips stacked and your knees bent in front of you. Find the neutral position of your pelvis and lengthen your waist equally on both sides. Place both arms in front, in line with your breastbone. Gently engage your centre.

Breathe in to prepare. Breathe out as you float your top arm up to the ceiling. Continue breathing out and rotate your upper back, allowing your head, neck and arm to follow the movement while keeping your pelvis still. Breathe in deeply as you hold the position. Breathe out and rotate your head, neck and upper back to return to the starting position. Allow your top arm to follow the movement before finishing by lowering this arm. Repeat up to 10 times on both sides.

THE PROGRAMME

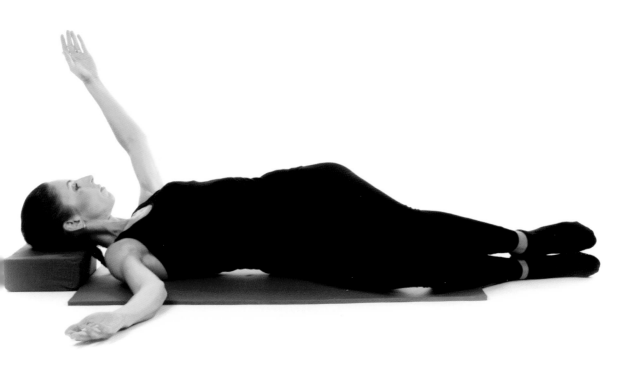

➤ To effectively mobilise your spine, focus your movement on the upper back and not on your arm. Once you have lifted your arm to vertical, there should be no more movement from the shoulder joint itself. Instead the arm should follow the movement of the ribcage and upper back.

➤ You may benefit from gently mobilising the nerves, which run from your neck through your arms. As you float your arm up, bend your wrist so that your palm faces upwards and hold this position throughout your movement. You may feel a mild tingling, which indicates that your nerves are positively responding to the stretch, but stop if you feel any pain.

➤ Maintain a gentle chin nod throughout, to prevent forward head posture.

➤ Maintain good alignment of your shoulder blade by gently gliding it downwards throughout the movement.

➤ Keep your arms and fingers long but avoid locking your elbow joints.

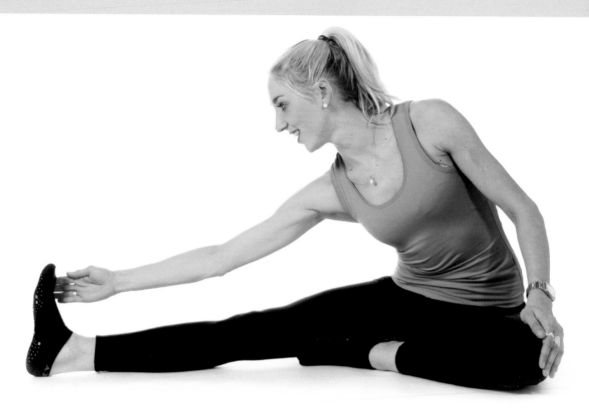

1. seated hamstring stretch

Promotes length and extensibility in your hamstring muscles and allows for greater freedom of your back and hip joints.

Sit with your right leg extended in front of you and your left leg bent. Align your pelvis and lower back into neutral, with even weight bearing through your sitting bones. Lengthen your spine upwards and engage your centre. Tilt your body towards your right leg until you feel a stretch down the back of your right thigh. Hold this stretch for up to 30 seconds and focus on lateral breathing.

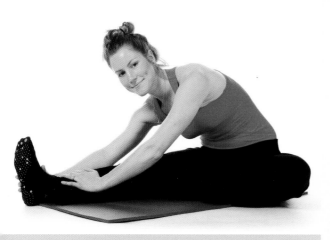

➤ If you have difficulty sitting comfortably, start by sitting on a small foam block, or step, until your lower back and hips become more mobile.

➤ You may benefit from mobilising the nerves that run from your spine down the back of your legs. Gently draw your foot back towards your body. A mild tingling will indicate that your nerves are positively responding to the stretch, but stop if you feel any pain. Hold this stretch for two seconds only. Repeat 10–15 times on each leg.

➤ Maintain the neutral spine position as you tilt your body forwards.

A mild tingling will indicate that your nerves are positively responding to the stretch.

2. lying nerve stretch

Promotes free gliding of the sciatic nerve between the interfacing muscles and connective tissues of the back of your leg.

Lie in the Pilates rest position. Gently engage your centre. Bend one leg into your chest and support the back of this thigh with both hands. Slowly straighten your knee as far as is comfortable. Hold this stretch for two seconds only. Stop if you feel any pain. Repeat 10–15 times on each leg.

➤ Do not flatten your lower back into the mat; instead maintain the neutral alignment.

➤ Avoid poking your chin forwards by keeping the back of your neck long.

➤ Avoid pulling through the arms – they are there to offer support for the leg.

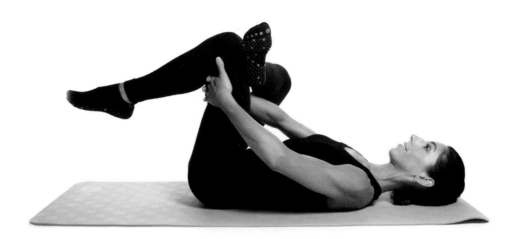

3. gluteal stretch

Encourages flexibility of the deep gluteal muscles to enhance mobility of your hips, pelvis and lower back.

Lie in the Pilates rest position and gently engage your centre. Cross your right leg onto the front of your left thigh and allow your right hip and knee to open outwards. Link your hands around the back of your left thigh and lift this leg into your chest. Hold this stretch for up to 30 seconds. Stop if you feel pain. Repeat 3–5 times on each leg.

HELP FROM THE PHYSIO

➤ You can use a wall for support. Lift your foot from the mat and place it flat onto a wall in front of you. Keep your back in the neutral spine position and support with your centre.

➤ If you still feel tight then spiky massage balls are great for releasing and loosening muscles. Place one underneath each buttock, then gently roll your buttock muscles side to side, up and down and then in circles.

➤ Keep a neutral spine position and your centre engaged to support your lower back throughout stretching.

➤ Do not pull with your arms when supporting your leg. Imagine your collarbones widening and the back of your neck lengthening to maintain good form.

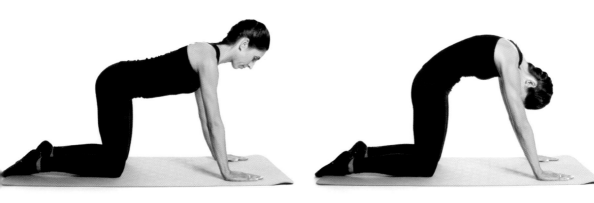

4. cat stretch

Trains sequential spinal mobilisation for greater freedom of movement and release of muscular tension throughout the day.

Move onto all fours on the mat. Place your hands slightly forwards of your shoulders and your knees directly under your hips. Lengthen your neck and spine into the neutral position. Lift your breastbone away from the mat to stabilise your shoulder blades. Gently engage your centre. Breathe in to prepare. Breathe out as you sequentially curve your spine into a C shape beginning with your tailbone and finishing with the crown of your head. Breathe in and maintain this position. Breathe out and sequentially elongate your spine from the tailbone to the crown of the head back into the neutral starting position. Repeat 3–5 times.

Slow and controlled movements will help to ensure you do not move your spine as a block.

5. hip flexor stretch

Counters the shortening effects of sitting and lengthens the muscles at the front of the hip joints.

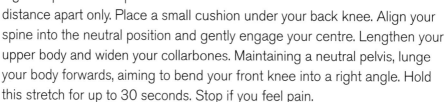

Come into a lunge position with a wall beside you for support. Ensure that the legs are positioned hip distance apart only. Place a small cushion under your back knee. Align your spine into the neutral position and gently engage your centre. Lengthen your upper body and widen your collarbones. Maintaining a neutral pelvis, lunge your body forwards, aiming to bend your front knee into a right angle. Hold this stretch for up to 30 seconds. Stop if you feel pain.

Repeat 3–5 times on each leg.

HELP FROM THE PHYSIO

➤ Tightness in the hip flexor muscles is common. Think of tucking your tailbone downwards to avoid arching your back.

➤ Do not bend your front knee beyond a right angle as this may place stress through the joint.

A tightness in the hip flexor muscles is common.

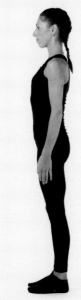
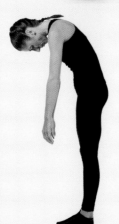
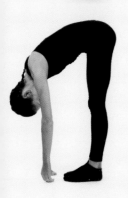

6. roll down

Promotes sequential and fluid mobility of the spine while encouraging accurate body awareness and posture in standing.

Stand with your upper back, shoulder blades and head resting against a wall. Keep your head and neck upright and lengthen the back of your neck. Position your feet approximately a foot's length away from the wall, hip distance apart, and bend your knees slightly. Position your spine in neutral alignment. Glide your shoulder blades downwards and relax your arms down long beside your body. Gently engage your centre.

Breathe in to prepare. Breathe out, nod your head and neck forwards and continue sequentially peeling your entire spine away from the wall. Allow the lower back to gently flatten into the wall before also rolling forwards. Keep your head and arms free and relaxed. Once you have rolled down as far as you can, breathe in wide to hold. Breathe out as you roll your pelvis back into the wall and continue sequentially rolling your entire spine until you are standing upright.

HELP FROM THE PHYSIO

➤ This movement mobilises your spine and the nerves that originate from your lower back and extend to your toes. Aim for a smooth and controlled roll of your spine.

➤ Aim for a deep C shape of your spine by rolling slowly through each section of your back. Your spine should roll directly forwards.

➤ Keep your knees slightly bent throughout the movement.

back to life
Centring in Everyday Life

Once you have learnt to connect with your centre, you can achieve greater confidence and freedom of movement in 'real' life by regular practice throughout the day.

1. hundreds in standing

Practise this every time you wash your hands, taking a few moments afterwards to align your body and engage your centre whilst standing.

Stand with your feet hip distance apart and your weight balanced evenly through the key points of your feet. Position your shoulders directly over your hips. Widen your collarbones, keeping your ribcage soft, and lengthen your entire spine.

To find your neutral spine position, imagine your pelvis as a bowl. Place your hands onto the brim of this bowl or around your waist and tilt your pelvic 'bowl' forwards and backwards. Repeat this a few times to achieve a smooth and controlled movement. Move your pelvic 'bowl' into an upright position where no water will spill. In this position, there should be a small, inwards curve of your lower back.

Now you are standing in good alignment, focus on a gentle connection with your deep centring muscles. Once you have found this connection, practise holding it while breathing naturally.

2. hundreds in sitting

Treat mealtimes as your daily practice sessions.

Sit on a chair with your feet hip distance apart. Ensure even weight-bearing through your sitting bones. Position your shoulders directly over your hips. Widen your collarbones, keeping your ribcage soft, and lengthen your spine.

Now imagine that your pelvis is a bowl. Place your hands onto the brim of this bowl or around your waist. Tilt your pelvic 'bowl' forwards and imagine spilling water out of the front. Then tilt your pelvic 'bowl' backwards to spill water out of the back. Repeat this a few times, aiming to isolate the movement to your lower back and pelvis while keeping the rest of your body still.

To find your neutral spine position, align your 'bowl' upright where no water spills out the front or back. In the neutral position, there should be a small inwards curve of your lower back. In this position, you may already feel some of your key abdominal stabilising muscles.

To be sure you are working effectively to maintain your neutral position, slowly engage your centre. Concentrate on a continuous connection with your centring muscles as you breathe normally.

WEEK ONE Checklist:

✓ 1. I can engage my Pilates centre when lying on my back.

✓ 2. I can control the neutral spine position when moving my leg along the floor.

✓ 3. There is no worsening of pain when my back moves during the shoulder bridge or arm openings exercises.

✓ 4. I have been practising aligning my body and centring whilst sitting to eat and standing to wash my hands.

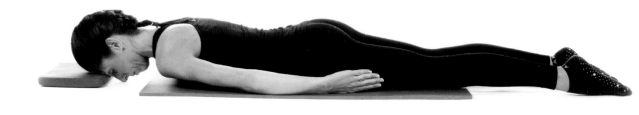

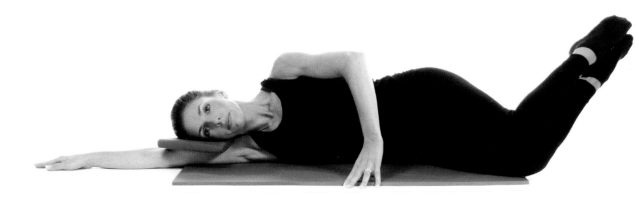

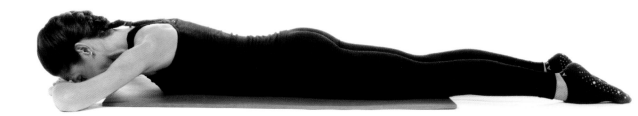

week 2

. . . the movements from week 1 now comprise your **Warm Up** and **Cool Down**.

Do not be tempted to skip the **Warm Up**. Correct activation of your centre is crucial to the success of your Pilates programme, and especially vital if you have back pain. The **Cool Down** will ensure that your body is in peak condition and ready for the rest of your day.

the warm up

- ✓ hundreds — *level one*
- ✓ one leg stretch — *level one*
- ✓ double leg stretch — *level one*
- ✓ the clam — *level one*
- ✓ hip twist — *level one*
- ✓ shoulder bridge — *level one*
- ✓ arm openings

the exercises

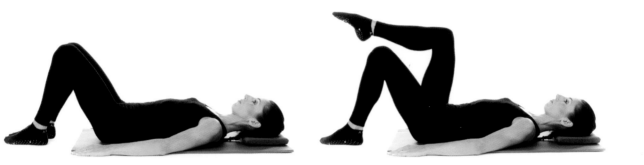

1. scissors *(level one)*

Challenges dynamic stability of your lower back and
pelvis during coordinated movement of your legs.

Lie in the Pilates rest position. Gently engage your centre. Breathe in to
prepare. Breathe out as you float one leg into the 'tabletop' position, where
your hip and knee are bent to right angles. Breathe in and hold. Breathe out
as you lower your leg. Repeat up to 10 times, alternating legs.

HELP FROM THE PHYSIO

➤ To check for correct abdominal muscle action, place one hand below your belly button.
As your leg lifts, the muscles under your hand should remain flat and not bulge or dome
forwards. This indicates a good connection with your centre.

➤ If the abdominal muscles dome forwards, start the movement by sliding your foot inwards
along the mat towards your sitting bone and then float the leg up, keeping the knee relaxed.
Then simply lower the leg to the mat.

➤ To prevent your pelvis from rocking, imagine balancing a tray of drinks on your lower
abdominal area.

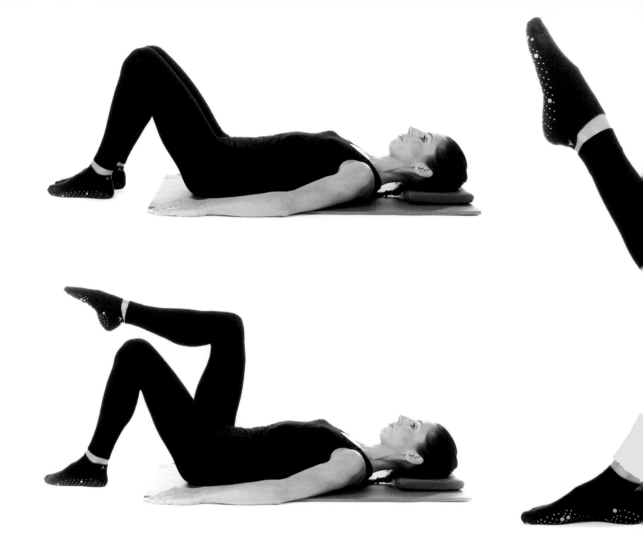

2. one leg stretch *(level two)*

Trains stability of your lower back and pelvis during coordinated movement of your legs.

Lie in the Pilates rest position. Gently engage your centre. Breathe in to prepare. Breathe out as you float one leg into the tabletop position. Breathe in and hold the position. Breathe out and extend your leg forwards and upwards on a diagonal line, maintaining neutral spine alignment. Breathe in and fold your leg back into the tabletop position. Breathe out and lower your leg. Repeat up to 10 times, alternating legs.

If you experience a clicking sensation at the front or side of your hip, it may indicate that your gluteal muscles are not working effectively.

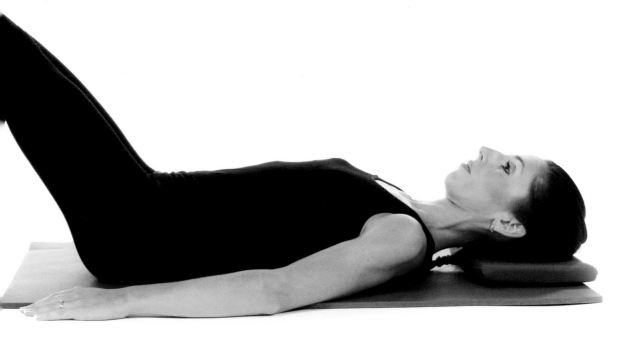

➤ If you experience a clicking sensation at the front or side of your hip, it may indicate that your gluteal muscles are not working effectively. To help engage these muscles, gently draw your sitting bones together as you extend your leg forwards.

➤ If you still experience clicking or clunking, loop a Pilates band under the sole of your foot and stretch your leg into the band as you extend your leg forwards. This will help to compress your hip and pelvic joints to support the weight of your leg.

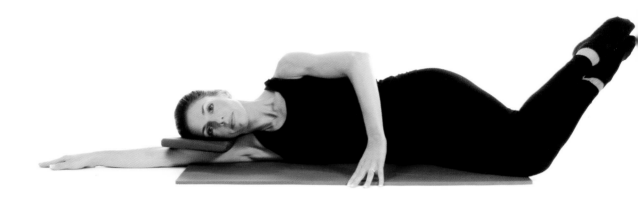

3. the clam *(level two)*

Isolates and strengthens the deep stabilising muscles of your hip and pelvis to create a more stable base of support. Start by practising level 1 (see page 59) and add level 2 to further strengthen your deep gluteal muscles through a larger movement.

Lie on one side with your hips and shoulders stacked, your knees bent and your thighs just forwards of your body, and then lift your feet up off the mat. Find the neutral position of your pelvis and lengthen your waist equally on both sides. Keep your lower arm extended under your head and your top hand on the mat for light support. Place a small cushion under your head. Gently engage your centre.

Breathe in to prepare. Breathe out as you lift your top knee upwards, keeping the feet lifted and your pelvis still. Breathe in as you lower your top leg, keeping your feet lifted and your pelvis still.
Repeat up to 10 times.

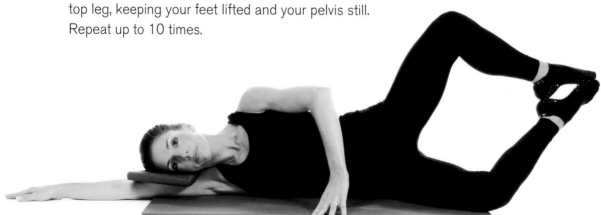

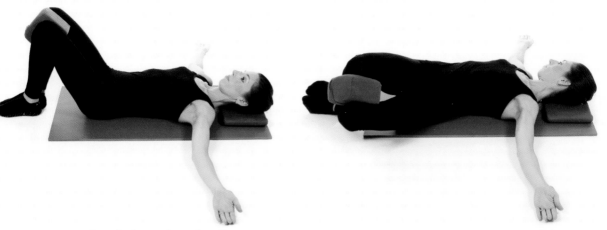

4. hip twist *(level two)*

Teaches controlled mobilisation of your back and pelvis while stabilising and opening the front of your chest and shoulders.

Lie in the Pilates rest position. Hold a small cushion between your knees and place the inner edges of your feet together. Position your arms out to the sides of your body, just below shoulder height, with your palms facing upwards. Gently engage your centre.

Breathe in to prepare. Breathe out as you sequentially roll your knees, pelvis and lower back to the left. Allow the right side of your pelvis and lower back to peel off the mat. Rotate your head and neck towards your right shoulder, keeping the back of your neck long. Breathe in deeply and hold the position. Breathe out as you roll your head and neck back to the midline and then continue sequentially rolling your lower back, pelvis and legs to the starting position. Repeat up to 10 times, alternating sides.

Keep your shoulder blades connected to the mat throughout the movement.

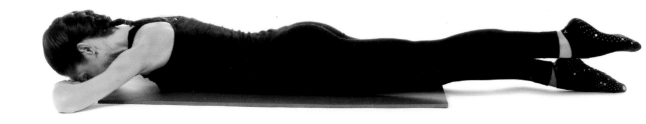

5. swimming *(level one)*

Strengthens your back and gluteal muscles through independent movement of your shoulders and hips to build control and stability of your pelvis.

Lie on your front with your legs hip distance apart and in parallel. Rest your forehead on the back of your hands. Lengthen the back of your neck and glide your shoulder blades downwards. Align your lower back into neutral. Gently engage your centre.

Breathe in to prepare. Breathe out as you lengthen and lift your left leg away from the mat. Breathe in and lower your leg. Repeat up to 10 times, alternating legs.

HELP FROM THE PHYSIO

➤ If your back is arching or you notice that you stand with a large curve in your lower back, commence this exercise with a cushion or two under your pelvis for support. Remove the cushions as your back control improves.

➤ You should feel your gluteal muscles working during this movement. If not, draw your sitting bones together just prior to lifting your leg. Keep up this little trick until the gluteal muscles work automatically.

➤ Lift your leg only as far as you can while keeping a stable back and pelvis.

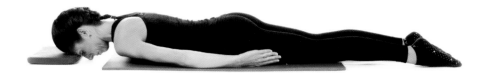

6. breaststroke prep *(level one)*

Promotes body awareness and stabilisation of
your head, neck and upper body, leading to a more
upright posture.

Lie on your front with your forehead resting on a small cushion, your arms
beside your body, your palms facing downwards and your legs hip distance
apart. Lengthen the back of your neck and glide your shoulder blades
downwards. Align your lower back into neutral. Gently engage your centre.

Breathe in to prepare. Breathe out as you reach downwards through your
arms and hover them above the mat. Breathe in, keeping your arms and
shoulder blades stable. Breathe out as you relax your shoulder blades and
lower your arms to the mat. Repeat up to 10 times.

HELP FROM THE PHYSIO

➤ Focus on movement and control of your shoulder blades rather than your arms. Keep
your collarbones wide and visualise your shoulder blades tracing a small 'V' shape on
your upper back.

➤ Do not lift your head from the cushion. Instead, focus on keeping the back of your
neck long.

➤ Reach and hover your arms a few inches from the mat only.

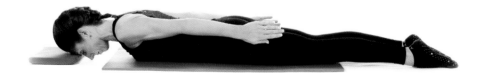

the cool down

- ✓ seated hamstring stretch
- ✓ lying nerve stretch
- ✓ gluteal stretch
- ✓ cat stretch
- ✓ hip flexor stretch
- ✓ roll down

back to life

Pacing and Chronic Pain

Fear of pain, resulting in avoidance of activity and exercise, can be a major obstacle to recovery for those with lower back pain. You may relate to the 'all or nothing' approach to exercise.

For example, this is when someone with chronic pain feels that they are having a good day and decides uncharacteristically to walk to the shops, spend an afternoon gardening followed by several hours' cooking. The next day, the worsening pain is blamed on the activities of the previous day, which are subsequently avoided. Over the next few weeks of inactivity and avoidance the pain settles, only for the cycle to repeat itself the next time the sufferer is having a 'good day'. The baseline level of general activity and fitness thus never improves.

'Pacing' skills are useful for breaking this kind of cycle. Pacing helps to identify realistic activity levels and teaches how to sensibly increase these to improve overall fitness while avoiding painful episodes. With the help of your physiotherapist, or your doctor if necessary, begin by establishing your baseline, or the amount of activity that you can do before your pain flares up. Whilst your baseline may be small to begin with, the important thing is that it can be developed over time to result in significant differences.

Chronic pain is a multifaceted syndrome and there are likely to be setbacks along the way. However, continue your realistic and progressive movement when it comes to activity and exercise, and you will feel the ultimate benefits over time.

Be patient! Small but steady steps will send you in the right direction towards recovery and a better quality of life.

WEEK TWO Checklist:

✓ 1. I can engage my Pilates centre when lying on my side.

✓ 2. I can engage my Pilates centre when lying on my front.

✓ 3. I am able to stretch in a controlled and comfortable manner.

✓ 4. I am gradually increasing my general activity and exercise through 'pacing'.

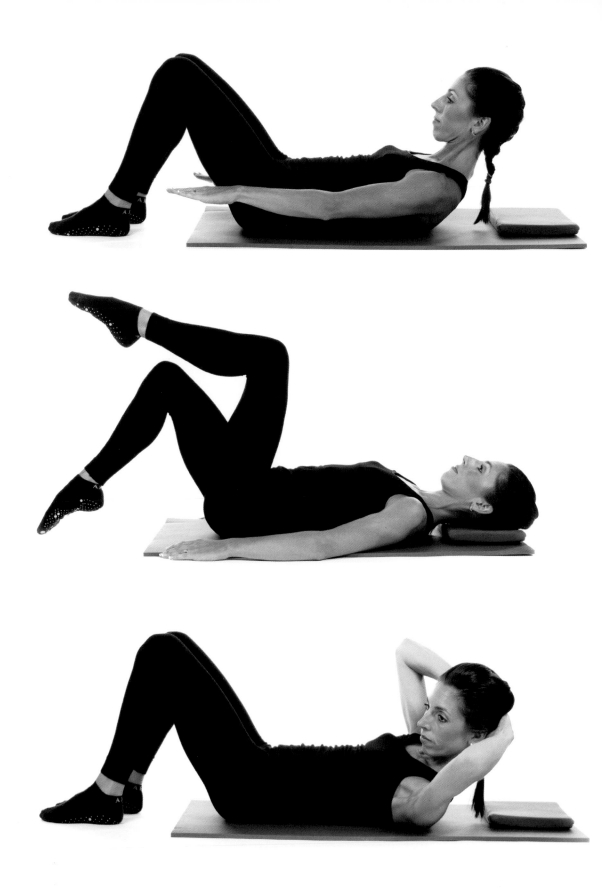

week 3

the warm up

✓	hundreds	*level one*
✓	one leg stretch	*level one*
✓	double leg stretch	*level one*
✓	the clam	*level one*
✓	hip twist	*level one*
✓	shoulder bridge	*level one*
✓	arm openings	

the exercises

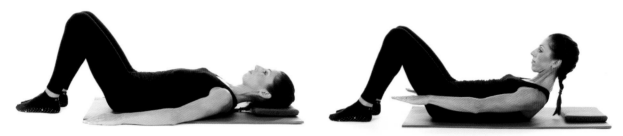

1. abdominal prep

Trains balance and strength of the abdominal muscles
to enable controlled movement of your spine and ribcage.

Lie in the Pilates rest position. Gently engage your centre. Breathe in to
prepare. Breathe out as you nod your chin downwards and sequentially
curl your head, neck, shoulders and upper back forwards off the mat.
Simultaneously, slide your shoulder blades downwards and raise your arms
to hover above the mat. Breathe in and maintain the position. Breathe out as
you sequentially lengthen and lower your upper body to the mat whilst also
lowering your arms to the mat. Repeat up to 10 times.

HELP FROM THE PHYSIO

➤ Neck discomfort? Start by practising with one or both hands supporting the back of your
head. Keep your elbows wide but within your peripheral vision and keep relaxing your
shoulder blades downwards.

➤ Do not flatten your lower back as you curl up. A thin cushion in the small of your back
will support the neutral spine position initially, if required.

➤ Support your pelvic floor! You should never feel a sense of bearing down with any Pilates
exercise. If unsure, gently squeeze your pelvic floor muscles to ensure good support.

THE PROGRAMME

2. oblique prep

Trains the abdominal muscles to enable controlled rotary movement of your spine and ribcage.

Lie in the Pilates rest position. Place your hands at the back of your head, with your elbows wide, just within your peripheral vision. Gently engage your centre. Breathe in to prepare. Breathe out as you nod your chin downwards and sequentially rotate your head, neck and upper body towards your left hip. Keep your pelvis level and your spine stable. Breathe out as you sequentially lengthen and lower the upper body back to the mat and into the midline starting position. Repeat up to 10 times, alternating sides.

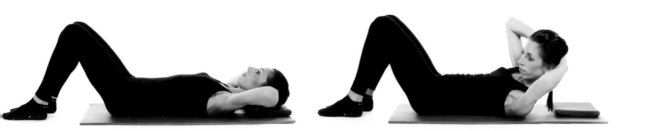

HELP FROM THE PHYSIO

➤ Maintain a gentle chin nod downwards throughout the movement.

➤ Do not flatten your lower back as you curl up. A thin cushion in the small of your back will support the neutral spine position initially, if required.

➤ Allow movement of your upper back only, and keep your pelvis and spine still.

➤ Avoid pulling forwards from your head, neck or shoulders.

➤ Avoid abdominal 'doming', which indicates a poor connection with your centre.

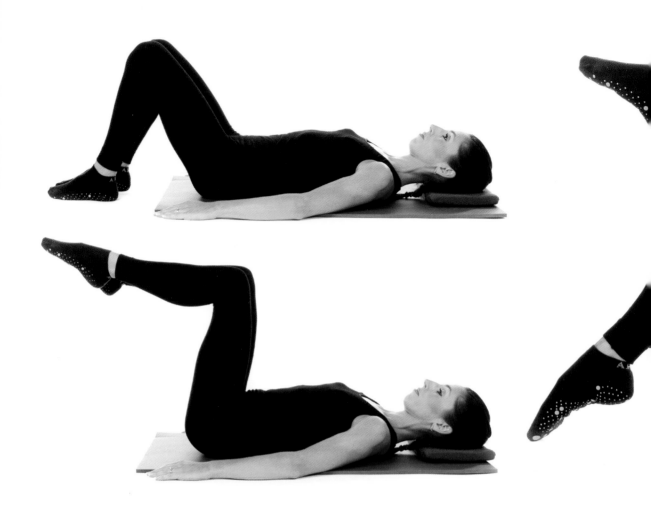

3. scissors *(level two)*

Strengthens your abdominal core while challenging dynamic stability of your lower back and pelvis during coordinated movement of your legs.

Lie in the Pilates rest position. Gently engage your centre. Breathe in to prepare. Breathe out as you float your right leg into the tabletop position. Breathe in and hold. Breathe out as you float your left leg into the tabletop position. Breathe in and check your centre and your neutral spine alignment. Breathe out as you lower one leg to tap the toes to the mat. Breathe in and float your leg back into the tabletop position. Repeat up to 10 times, alternating legs. To finish, breathe out and lower one leg at a time.

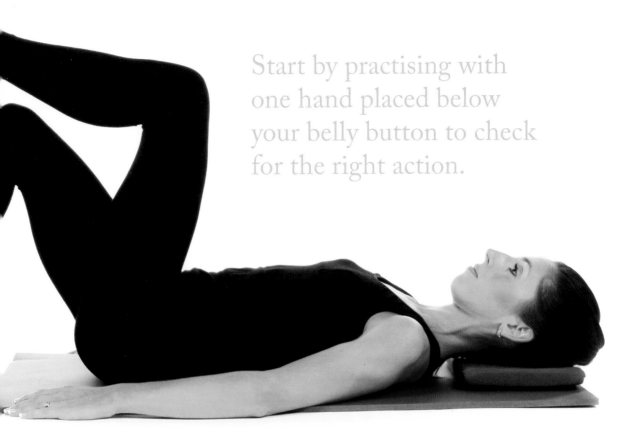

Start by practising with
one hand placed below
your belly button to check
for the right action.

➤ Start by practising with one hand placed below your belly button to check for the right action. As your leg lifts, the muscles under your hand should remain flat and not bulge or dome forwards.

➤ If you feel abdominal doming, start with 'mini leg' scissors: in the double tabletop position, allow your knees to fully bend so that the back of your thighs and calf muscles touch. Practise the movement, keeping the knees fully bent so that you are effectively working with a shorter lever arm and less load on your spine.

➤ Do not arch your back as your foot lowers to tap the mat.

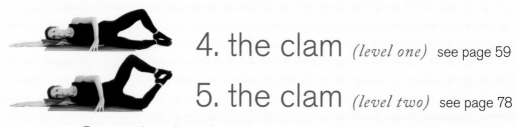

4. the clam *(level one)* see page 59

5. the clam *(level two)* see page 78

6. side kick

Strengthens the deep hip and pelvic stabilising muscles while challenging control, balance and coordination.

Lie on one side with your hips and shoulders stacked, your legs extended slightly in front of your body and your feet flexed. Find the neutral position of your pelvis and lengthen your waist equally on both sides. Keep your lower arm extended under your head and your top hand on the mat for light support. Place a small cushion under your head. Gently engage your centre.

Breathe in to prepare. Breathe out and lift your top leg to hip height, then reach this leg forwards as far as you can while keeping your pelvis and spine stable. As your leg glides forwards, point your foot and ankle. Breathe in and glide your leg back, keeping it lifted at hip height. As your leg glides backwards, flex your foot and ankle. Repeat up to 10 times on one side and then repeat on the opposite side.

HELP FROM THE PHYSIO

➤ Difficulty balancing? Start with your bottom knee bent to create a more stable base. Return to the more challenging position as your balance improves.

➤ Don't be tempted to move your leg too far forwards or backwards. The movement is determined by your joint mobility and muscle flexibility as well as your pelvic stability. Start with small movements and progress as you improve.

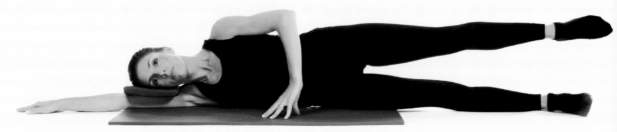

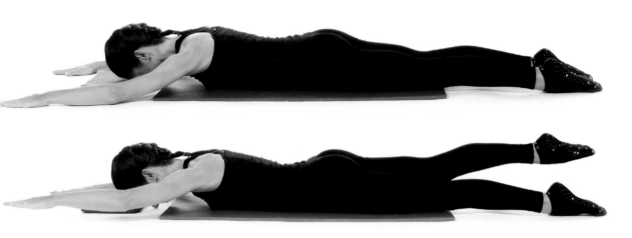

7. swimming *(level one)* see page 80

8. swimming progression

Strengthens your back and gluteal muscles through independent movement of your shoulders and hips to achieve control and stability of the pelvis.

Lie on your front with your legs hip distance apart. Rest your forehead on a small cushion. Place your arms overhead with your hands slightly wider than shoulder width. Lengthen the back of your neck and glide your shoulder blades downwards. Align your lower back into neutral. Gently engage your centre.

Breathe in to prepare. Breathe out as you lengthen and lift your left arm and right leg away from the mat. Breathe in and lower this arm and leg to the mat. Repeat up to 10 times, alternating with opposite arms and legs.

If you have a forwards curve of your upper back (termed a 'kyphosis'), continue practising with leg lifts only.

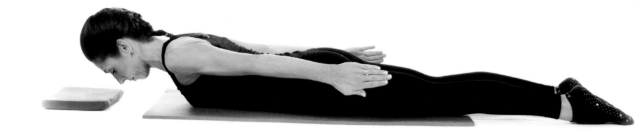

9. breaststroke prep progression

Promotes body awareness and stabilisation of your head, neck and upper body, leading to a more upright posture.

Lie on your front with your forehead resting on a small cushion, your arms resting beside your body, your palms facing inwards and your legs hip distance apart. Lengthen the back of your neck and glide your shoulder blades downwards. Align your lower back into neutral. Gently engage your centre.

Breathe in to prepare. Breathe out as you lengthen and lift your head, neck and upper body away from the mat. Simultaneously, reach and lift your arms so that they hover above the mat. Breathe in, keeping your upper body stable. Breathe out as you lower your upper body and arms to the mat. Repeat up to 10 times.

HELP FROM THE PHYSIO

➤ Maintain a gentle chin nod throughout the movement.

➤ To train better upper body posture, focus on movement and control of your upper body and shoulder blades rather than your arms.

➤ Keep your collarbones wide and visualise your shoulder blades tracing a small V shape on your upper back.

➤ Use one or two pillows under your pelvis to help prevent your lower back from arching initially, if required.

10. spine twist

Promotes healthy posture and position awareness in sitting whilst strengthening the abdominal muscles to produce spinal rotation.

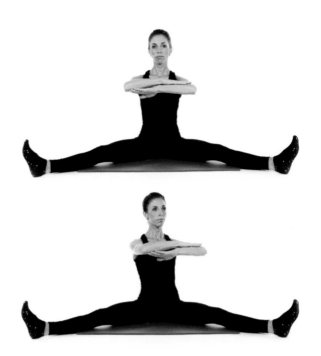

Sit on a chair with your feet hip distance apart or sit comfortably on the mat. Position your pelvis into neutral and lengthen your spine upwards. Fold your arms on top of each other and lift them in front of your breastbone. Keeping your ribcage soft, slide your shoulder blades gently downwards into a V shape on your upper back. Gently engage your centre.

Breathe in to prepare. Breathe out as you twist your body to the left, keeping your lower back and pelvis stable. Imagine growing taller from your waist as you twist. Breathe in wide to the sides and back of the ribcage. Breathe out as you twist your body back to the centre, maintaining a lengthened spine. Repeat up to 10 times, alternating sides.

HELP FROM THE PHYSIO

➤ To effectively mobilise your upper back, keep your pelvis and lower back still. Imagine your sitting bones are anchors to prevent any movement of your pelvis.

➤ Don't cheat by stealing movement from your neck and arms. Imagine holding a beach ball against your breastbone to help keep your arms still.

➤ Keep your nose in line with your breastbone to prevent excessive neck movement.

➤ Make sure you don't tip your body sideways as it twists. Think of keeping your waist equally long on both sides.

➤ Relax your shoulder blades downwards throughout the movement.

the cool down

✓ seated hamstring stretch
✓ lying nerve stretch
✓ gluteal stretch
✓ cat stretch
✓ hip flexor stretch
✓ roll down

back to life

Stop Sitting for so Long!

Up to 9 out of 10 adults suffer from back pain at some point in life and, according to one recent report, 5 out of 10 working adults have back pain every year. Not surprising when you consider that most of us spend the greater part of our day – a spectacular 14 hours and 39 minutes, if you're British! – sitting down.

If you lead a sedentary lifestyle (think about your day, and the amount of time you spend off your feet, working at the computer, commuting, eating, drinking, and relaxing in front of the TV), you will undoubtedly suffer from poor posture, most commonly referred to as forward head posture, which causes headaches and shoulder and back pain. For every inch of forward head tilt beyond the norm, the neck experiences up to an extra 10 pounds of load. Over long periods of time, this can lead to sprains and injuries on the neck and back. In the longer term, it can lead to injuries to the joints, discs and spinal chord itself.

A simple yet challenging task for this week is to avoid staying in any position for longer than 10 minutes. To ensure success, here are some tips:

- If travelling for long periods on public transport, alternate sitting and standing every 10 minutes.

- If working at a desk for long periods, set Outlook to flash up every 10 minutes, reminding you to stand, stretch or take a short walk around the office or home.

- Encourage active socialising with friends. Instead of sitting at a cafe for coffee, take a stroll instead.

- Limit television in the evening and stand for every advertisement to change your position.

- If reading in bed at night, alternate lying on your side with sitting and reclining, to ensure you move every 10 minutes.

WEEK THREE Checklist:

✓ 1. My neck feels comfortable during the abdominal and oblique prep.

✓ 2. I can engage my Pilates centre during scissors (level two). If not, continue practising scissors (level one) for the next week. If you feel the correct activation but cannot hold it, it is likely that you are engaging your centre well but that it fatigues quickly. Continue with the double tabletop position but limit your repetitions.

✓ 3. I am making the effort to move frequently and sit less.

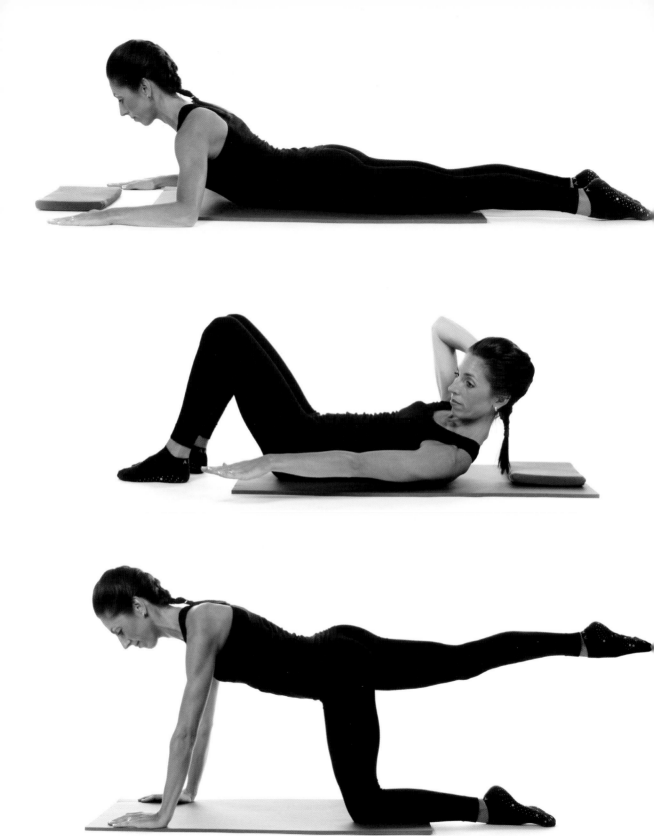

week 4

the warm up

- ✓ hundreds — *level one*
- ✓ one leg stretch — *level one*
- ✓ double leg stretch — *level one*
- ✓ the clam — *level one*
- ✓ hip twist — *level one*
- ✓ shoulder bridge — *level one*
- ✓ arm openings

the exercises

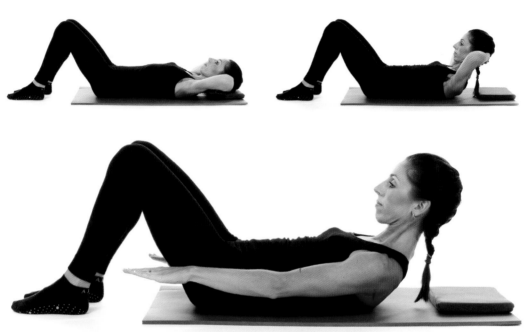

1. abdominal prep challenge

Trains balance and strength of the abdominal muscles to enable controlled movement of your spine and ribcage.

Lie in the Pilates rest position. Place your hands at the back of your head, with your elbows wide, just within your peripheral vision. Gently engage your centre. Breathe in to prepare. Breathe out as you nod your chin and curl your head, neck, shoulders and upper body forwards off the mat. Breathe in, keeping your upper body scooped, reach both arms forwards and hover them above the mat. Breathe out, place your hands at the back of your head, still keeping your upper body scooped. Breathe in as you sequentially lengthen and lower your upper body to the mat. Repeat up to 10 times.

THE PROGRAMME

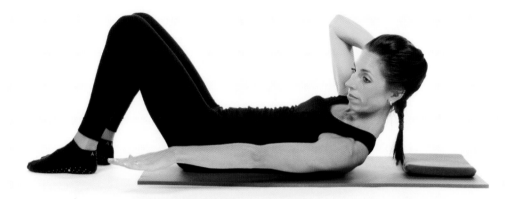

2. oblique prep challenge

Trains balance and strength of the abdominal muscles to enable controlled rotary movement of your spine and ribcage.

Lie in the Pilates rest position. Place your hands at the back of your head, with your elbows wide, just within your peripheral vision. Gently engage your centre. Breathe in to prepare. Breathe out as you nod your chin downwards and sequentially rotate your head, neck and upper body towards your left hip. Keep your pelvis level and your spine stable. Breathe in, keeping your upper body rotated, and reach your left arm forwards to hover above the mat. Breathe out, place your hand at the back of your head, still keeping your upper body rotated. Breathe in as you sequentially lengthen and lower the upper body to the centre of your mat. Repeat up to 10 times, alternating sides.

HELP FROM THE PHYSIO

➤ Support your head with your hands if required and hold your abdominal or oblique prep position for a pause as you take a full breath before lowering to the mat again.

➤ Keep your elbows wide but within your peripheral vision and do not hitch your shoulder blades upwards.

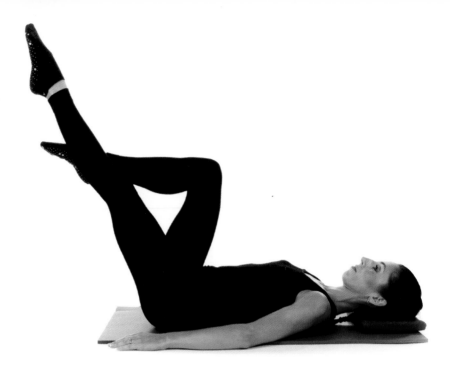

3. one leg stretch *(level three)*

Trains stability of your lower back and pelvis during coordinated movement of your legs.

Lie in the Pilates rest position. Gently engage your centre and then lift one leg at a time into the tabletop position. Breathe in to prepare. Breathe out as you extend your right leg forwards and upwards on a diagonal line, maintaining the neutral spine position. Breathe in as you fold your leg back into the tabletop position. Continue alternating legs up to 10 times. To finish, lower your legs to the mat one at a time.

HELP FROM THE PHYSIO

➤ Engage your deep gluteal muscles as you extend your leg, to avoid clicking or tension at the front of your hip. If you do experience a clicking sensation, practise with your Pilates band looped under the sole of one foot. Then swap the band over and repeat on the opposite leg.

➤ To train the sensation around your hip and knee, practise this exercise with a Swiss Ball positioned under the soles of your feet – the multi-directional, unstable surface will teach you control.

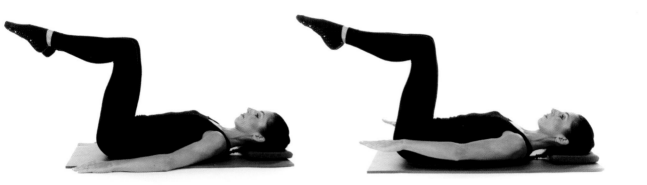

4. hundreds *(level two)*

Combines endurance training of the abdominal 'centre' with lateral breathing and accurate body alignment.

Lie in the Pilates rest position. Gently engage your centre and then lift one leg at a time into the tabletop position. Breathe in and check that you remain in neutral spine alignment with your centre engaged. Breathe out for 5 counts as you beat your arms up and down in a small, sharp movement 5 times. Breathe in for 5 counts, beating your arms up and down 5 times. Repeat up to 10 times to reach 100 beats. To finish, slowly lower your legs to the mat one at a time as you breathe out.

HELP FROM THE PHYSIO

➤ Hundreds is a great endurance challenge. However, if you do tire, lower one leg to the mat and continue beating with your arms. With routine practice, you will build the endurance required for the ultimate 100!

➤ With the hundreds breathing, aim to time your downward arm beat on a breath out, then take a short, quick breath in, ready for your next downward arm beat as you breathe out. If you find that there is too much to think about in the beginning, focus on normal lateral breathing.

➤ Avoid abdominal doming by focusing on your deep abdominals and pelvic floor muscles. Keep your arms lengthening forwards but do not lock your elbow joints.

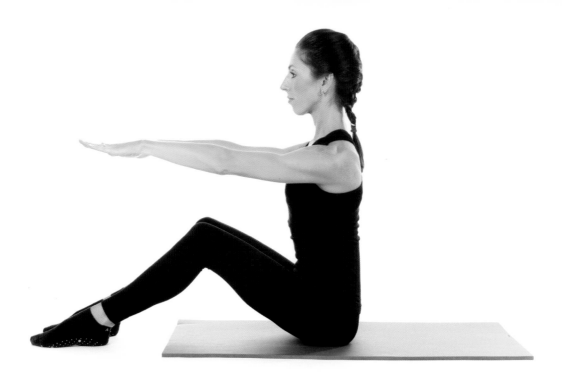

5. roll up

Promotes healthy posture and position awareness
in sitting whilst also creating a fluid spine through
sequential mobilisation.

Sit on a chair or on your mat with your legs in front, hip distance apart,
and your knees bent slightly. Align your pelvis into the neutral position and
lengthen your spine upwards. Lift your arms forwards to shoulder height
with your palms facing downwards. Slide your shoulder blades gently
downwards into a V shape on your upper back. Gently engage your centre.

Breathe in to prepare. Breathe out as you roll your tailbone and pelvis
backwards and sequentially round your lower and mid back into a C shape.
Keep your arms lifted forwards and your head upright. Breathe in wide,
maintaining your C shape. Breathe out as you roll your C shaped body
forwards over your hips and then sequentially lengthen your spine upwards.
Repeat up to 10 times.

THE PROGRAMME

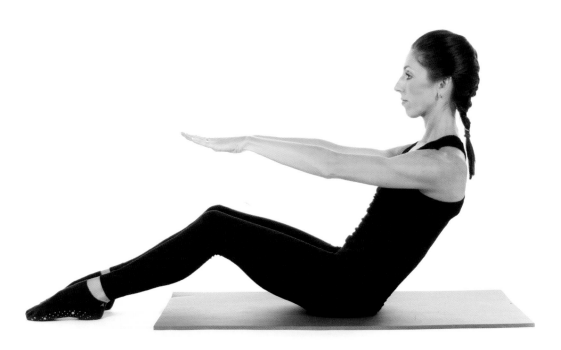

➤ Imagine that your pelvis is a wheel rolling backwards to create a roundness in your lower back.

➤ Imagine there is a harness around your middle, which is attached to a pulley behind you. The pulley is trying to draw your waist backwards and your upper body and sitting bones are resisting its movement.

➤ Roll back only as far as you can with a C shape to your spine to avoid strain on your lower back.

➤ Draw your lower abdominals in deep as you curve your spine.

➤ Keep your upper body broad and your head and neck upright as you create your curve. Imagine balancing a book on the top of your head.

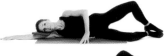 6. the clam *(level one)* see page 59

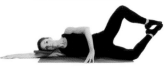 7. the clam *(level two)* see page 78

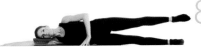 8. side kick see page 90

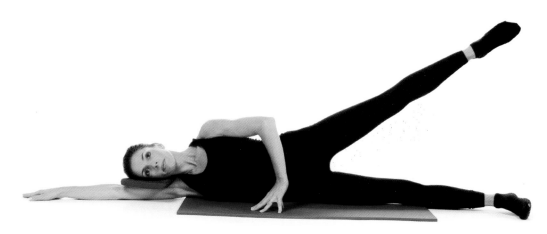

9. side leg lift

Isolates and strengthens the deep stabilising muscles of your hip and pelvis and encourages length and tone of the leg.

Lie on one side with your hips and shoulders stacked, your legs extended in line with your body and your feet flexed. Find the neutral position of your pelvis and lengthen your waist equally on both sides. Keep your lower arm extended under your head and your top hand on the mat for light support. Place a small cushion under your head. Gently engage your centre.

Breathe in to prepare. Breathe out as you reach and lift your top leg upwards. Breathe in and lower your leg to the height of your pelvis. Repeat up to 10 times and then repeat on the other side.

HELP FROM THE PHYSIO

➤   Difficulty balancing? Start with your bottom knee bent to create a more stable base. Return to the more challenging position as your balance improves.

➤   Keep the movement controlled and within the limits of your hip. Start with small movements and progress as your control improves.

➤   If your waist sinks into the mat as you lift your leg, start by placing a thin cushion under your waist.

THE PROGRAMME

10. swimming in four-point kneeling

Promotes pelvic and shoulder blade stability through the use of the body's muscular sling support system.

Move onto all fours on the mat. Place your hands slightly forwards of your shoulders, and your knees directly under your hips. Lengthen your neck and spine into the neutral position. Lift your breastbone away from the mat to stabilise your shoulder blades. Gently engage your centre.

Breathe in to prepare. Breathe out as you slide your right leg away and then raise it off the mat to hip height. Breathe in as you lower your leg to the mat. Repeat up to 10 times, alternating legs.

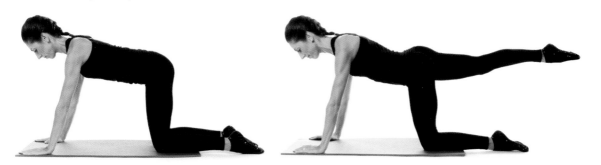

HELP FROM THE PHYSIO

➤ If your back arches as you lift your leg, start by keeping your foot on the mat. With routine practice, you can progressively lift your leg away from the mat.

➤ To learn good control, tie a small loop in one end of your Pilates band and place it around the sole of the moving foot. Hold the other end with your opposite hand. Practise the movement on one leg at a time.

➤ Keep your centre drawn inwards and if you have any knee discomfort, place a cushion under your knees.

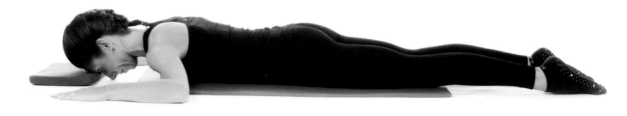

11. breastroke prep *(level two)*

Promotes body awareness and stabilisation of your head, neck and upper body, leading to a more upright posture.

Lie on your front with your forehead resting on a small cushion, your arms bent with your elbows just below shoulder height, and your legs hip distance apart. Lengthen the back of your neck and glide your shoulder blades downwards. Align your lower back into neutral. Gently engage your centre.

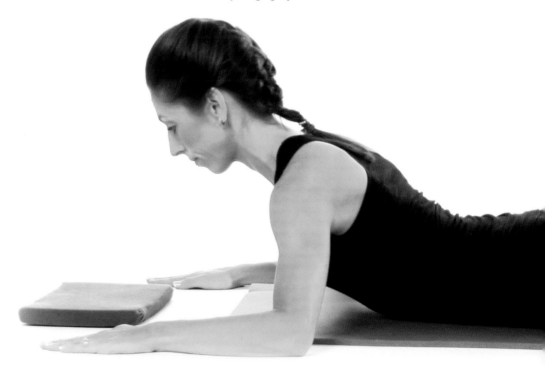

THE PROGRAMME

Breathe in to prepare. Breathe out as you sequentially lift your head, neck and upper body, keeping your arms on the mat. Keep lengthening the back of your neck and maintain neutral alignment of the lower back. Breathe in wide and hold the position. Breathe out as you lower your head, neck and upper body to the mat. Repeat up to 10 times.

HELP FROM THE PHYSIO

➤ Maintain a gentle chin nod throughout so as not to poke your chin forwards.

➤ Start with a cushion under your pelvis for support if required.

➤ Keep your movement small and focused on the upper spine only. There should be no movement of your lower back or lifting of your legs from the mat.

➤ Visualise your shoulder blades drawing a small V shape on your upper back and keep the collarbones wide.

Keep your movement small and focused on the upper spine only. There should be no movement of your lower back or lifting of your legs from the mat.

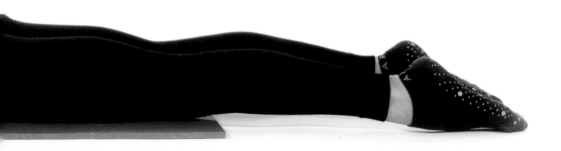

the cool down

- ✓ seated hamstring stretch
- ✓ lying nerve stretch
- ✓ gluteal stretch
- ✓ cat stretch
- ✓ hip flexor stretch
- ✓ roll down

back to life
The Work Environment

If you spend the bulk of your day sat down, your working environment may be contributing to your poor posture.

- Ensure that the back of your chair supports the natural curve in your lower back. The right office chair can help position the spine ideally and reduce muscle fatigue.

- Check that you have adequate leg room under your desk. Are you able to position your feet flat on the floor? If not, use a footrest and check that your hips and knees are bent at slightly greater than right angles.

- Place your keyboard and screen directly in front of you so that your shoulders are front-on to the computer. When typing, your upper arms should fall comfortably by your sides with your elbows bent slightly less than a right angle.

- Everything you need to access on your desk should be within reach and as close to your body as possible.

- Minimise eye strain by allowing an arm's length between your eyes and the screen. Position the top of your screen at approximately eye level. Use blinds to control sun glare.

- Keep your wrists straight whilst typing – don't bend them. You should type with your hands and wrists hovering just above the keyboard. Choose a flat mouse that fits the size of your hand and move it with your arm to avoid overuse, or bending of the wrist.

BREAK IT UP.
Change your posture
throughout your
workday, and take
regular breaks (every
10-15 minutes) to
help reduce overuse,
repetitive strain
injury and fatigue.

WEEK FOUR Checklist:

✓ **1.** I can actively isolate my deep Pilates core in any position.

✓ **2.** I can exercise in four-point kneeling without arching my back.

✓ **3.** I have considered my work environment and adjusted it to be more efficient.

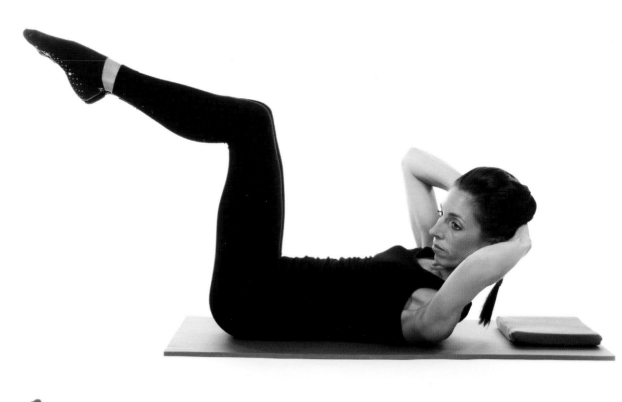

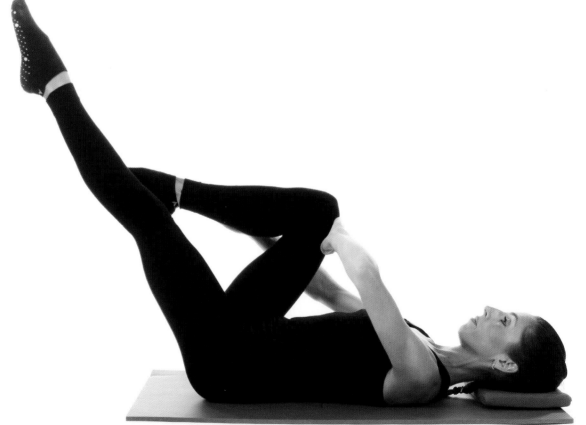

week 5

the warm up

- ✓ hundreds — *level one*
- ✓ one leg stretch — *level one*
- ✓ double leg stretch — *level one*
- ✓ the clam — *level one*
- ✓ hip twist — *level one*
- ✓ shoulder bridge — *level one*
- ✓ arm openings

the exercises

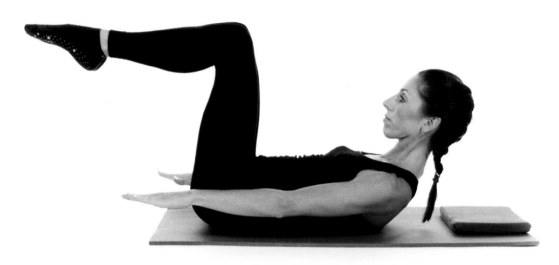

1. abdominal prep in tabletop

Trains balance and strength of the abdominal muscles to enable controlled movement of your spine and ribcage.

Lie in the Pilates rest position. Gently engage your centre and lift one leg into the tabletop position.

Breathe in to prepare. Breathe out as you nod your chin and sequentially curl your head, neck and upper back forwards off the mat while holding the tabletop position of your legs. At the same time, reach through your arms and hover them away from the mat. Breathe in wide and hold your abdominal preparation position. Breathe out as you lengthen and lower the upper body and arms to the mat while keeping your legs in the tabletop position. Repeat up to 10 times.

THE PROGRAMME

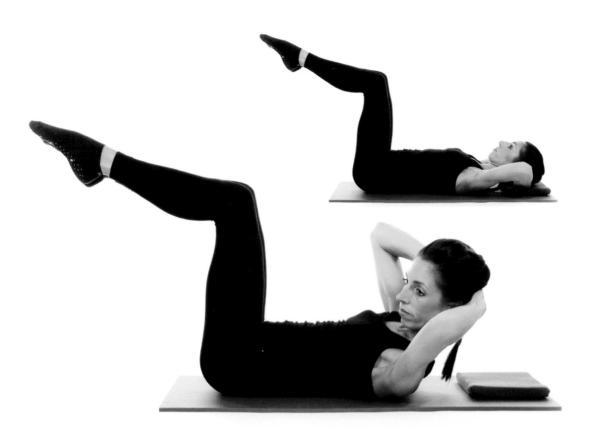

2. oblique prep in tabletop

Trains balance and strength of the abdominal muscles
to enable controlled rotary movement of your spine
and ribcage.

Lie in the Pilates rest position. Place your hands at the back of your head,
with your elbows wide, just within your peripheral vision. Gently engage
your centre and lift one leg at a time into the tabletop position.

Breathe in to prepare. Breathe out as you nod your chin downwards and
sequentially rotate your head, neck and upper body towards your left hip.
Breathe in as you lengthen and lower your upper body to the centre of
your mat. Repeat up to 10 times, alternating sides.

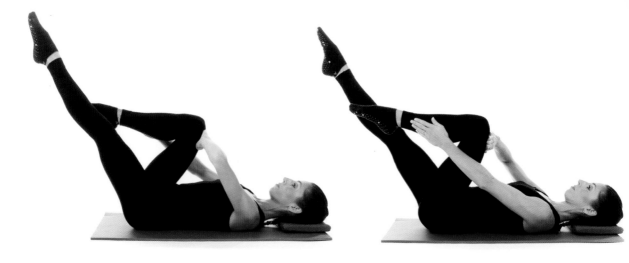

3. one leg stretch *(level four)*

Trains stability of your lower back and pelvis during coordinated movement of your legs.

Lie in the Pilates rest position. Gently engage your centre and lift one leg at a time into the tabletop position.

Breathe in to prepare. Breathe out as you extend your right leg forwards and upwards on a diagonal line. Simultaneously reach your left hand to the outside of your left lower leg and place your right hand across the top of your left knee. Take a short breath in. Breathe out as you return your right leg and extend your left leg forwards and upwards on a diagonal line. Simultaneously reach your right hand to the outside of your lower right leg and place your left hand across the top of your right knee.

Continue alternating legs and arms up to 10 times. Breathe out each time you extend your leg and take a short breath in as you alternate legs and arms. To finish, lower one leg at a time to your mat.

If you feel your back arching or bracing, spiky massage balls can help.

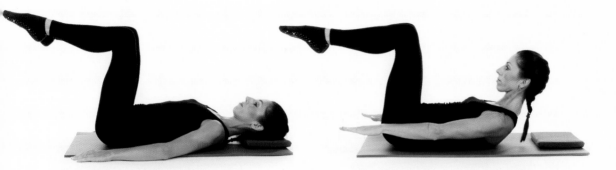

4. hundreds *(level three)*

Combines endurance training of the abdominal 'centre' with lateral breathing and accurate body alignment.

Lie in the Pilates rest position. Gently engage your centre and lift one leg at a time into the tabletop position. Breathe in to prepare. Breathe out as you curl your head, neck and upper body into the abdominal preparation position. Maintaining this position, breathe in for 5 counts as you beat your arms up and down in a small, sharp movement 5 times. Breathe out for 5 counts, beating your arms up and down 5 times. Repeat up to 10 times to reach 100 beats. To finish, lower your upper body to the mat and then lower your legs to the mat one at a time.

HELP FROM THE PHYSIO

➤ This is now an advanced movement. Support your head with one hand if required or lower your upper body to the mat if you cannot maintain good centring. Keep practising in the modified position until you build the control required for the ultimate 100!

➤ If you find that there is too much to think about, focus on normal lateral breathing and add the hundreds breathing once you have mastered your core.

➤ Maintain your gentle chin nod to avoid poor neck posture and strain. Look to your knees to help guide correct head and neck placement.

➤ Check that the movement of your arm beats originate from your shoulders only. Keep your arms lengthening forwards but do not lock your elbow joints.

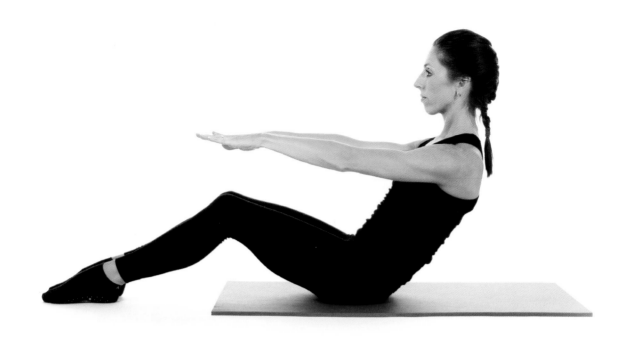

5. roll up see page 102
6. roll up with obliques

Promotes healthy posture and position awareness in sitting whilst also strengthening the oblique abdominal muscles to create effortless spinal movement.

Sit on your mat with your legs in front, hip distance apart, and your knees bent slightly. Align your pelvis into the neutral position and lengthen your spine upwards. Lift your arms forwards to shoulder height with your palms facing downwards. Slide your shoulder blades gently downwards into a V shape on your upper back. Gently engage your centre.

Breathe in to prepare. Breathe out as you roll your tailbone and pelvis backwards and sequentially round your lower and mid back into a C shape. Breathe in wide, maintaining the C shape of your spine. Breathe out, twist

THE PROGRAMME

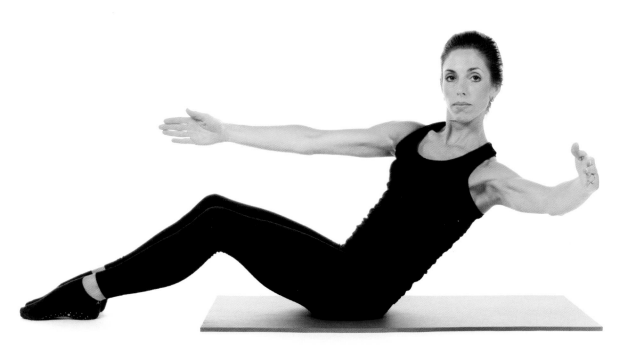

your upper body to the left, allowing your head and neck to follow the movement. Simultaneously, open your left arm to the side and keep your right arm reaching forwards. Breathe in, twist your upper body, head and neck back to the centre. Reach both arms forwards. Repeat on the opposite side. Repeat up to 10 times alternating sides. Finish by breathing out as you roll your C shaped spine forwards over your hips and then sequentially lengthen your spine upwards.

HELP FROM THE PHYSIO

➤ If your upper back is feeling stiff as you rotate, roll onto your side and practise a few repetitions of the arm openings exercise. Repeat on both sides and then return to the roll up with obliques exercise. Your spine should rotate more freely now.

➤ Keep your collarbones wide and your head and neck upright.

➤ Allow your arms, neck and head to follow the movement of your spine and move no further beyond this.

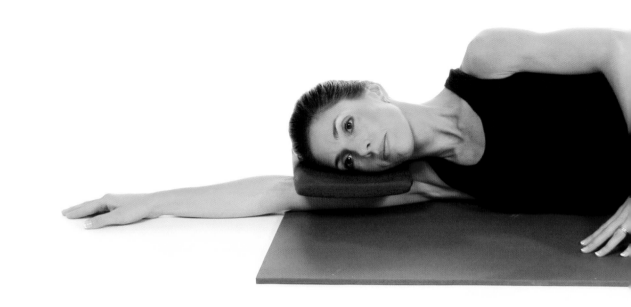

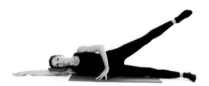

7. side kick see page 90

8. side leg lift see page 104

9. side leg circles

Isolates and strengthens the deep stabilising muscles of your hip and pelvis, encourages length and tone of the leg and mobilises the hip joint.

Lie on one side with your hips and shoulders stacked, your legs extended in line with your body and your feet flexed. Find the neutral position of your pelvis and lengthen your waist equally on both sides. Keep your lower arm extended under your head and your top hand on the mat for light support. Place a small cushion under your head. Gently engage your centre and then lift your top leg to hip height.

118

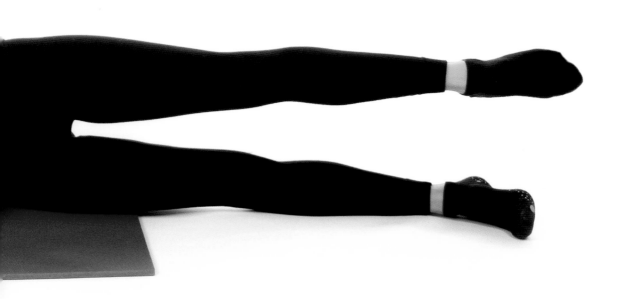

Breathe in to prepare. Breathe out as you circle your top leg outwards in a small circle. Take a short breath in as you return to the starting position. Repeat up to 10 times and then repeat 10 circles in the opposite direction. Repeat the series on your opposite side.

HELP FROM THE PHYSIO

➤ The degree of movement at your hip is determined by joint mobility, flexibility of muscles surrounding your hip as well as stability around your back and pelvis. Start small and progress as these elements improve.

➤ Often the outer thigh muscles dominate during this exercise rather than the better-suited gluteal muscles. If you are having difficulty feeling your gluteal muscles work, start by rotating your hip outwards so that your knee, ankle and toes face upwards. Maintain this hip rotation throughout your movements.

➤ If you feel that you are losing control of your position, start by practising with your bottom knee bent to create a more stable base. Return to the more challenging position as soon as you can.

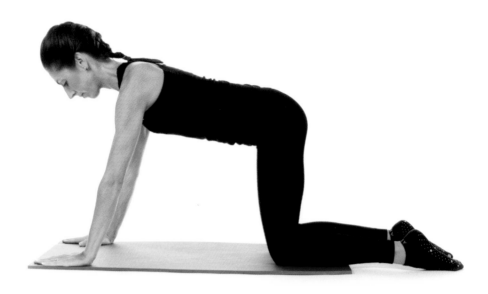

10. swimming in four-point kneeling progression

Promotes pelvic and shoulder blade stability through the use of the body's muscular sling support system.

Kneel on all fours with your hands slightly forwards of your shoulders and your knees directly under your hips. Lengthen and align the spine into neutral. Position your head and neck in line with your trunk. Keep your arms straight and gently lift your chest away from the mat to stabilise your shoulder blades. Gently engage your centre.

Breathe in to prepare. Breathe out as you slide and then lift your right leg away from the mat to hip height. At the same time, bring your left arm forwards to shoulder height. Breathe in as you lower the leg and arm to return to the starting position. Repeat up to 10 times alternating opposite arms and legs.

Avoid sideways rocking of your pelvis. Focus on keeping your pelvis level.

➤ If it feels difficult to raise your arm to shoulder height, start by lifting your hand to hover just above the mat. Slowly increase the height of your arm reach as your control improves.

➤ If you feel that you are arching or tilting your back when you lift your leg, start by keeping your foot in contact with the mat. With routine practice, begin to lift your leg in a small range and then progress until your leg can be lifted to hip height.

➤ For feedback about the level of engagement of your deep abdominal centre, release your centre and feel your abdominal wall sink towards the mat. Next, engage your centre and feel the movement of your abdominal wall as it correctly migrates towards the front of your spine. Aim to hold this position to keep the centre set through the movement.

➤ Whilst your shoulder blade will naturally move as you lift your arm, aim for a gentle downwards glide of your shoulder blade throughout the movement.

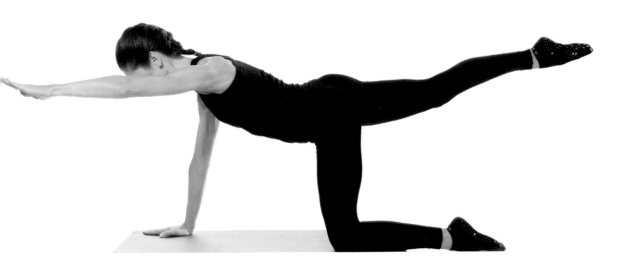

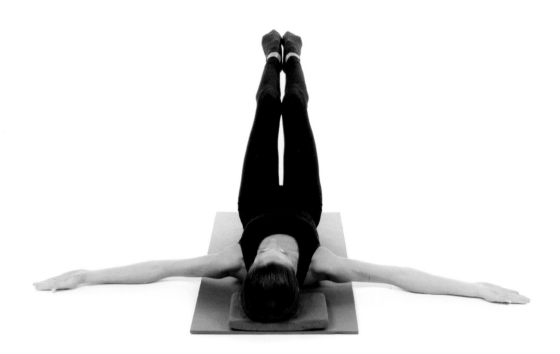

11. hip twist *(level four)*

Strengthens the oblique abdominal muscles to produce controlled and fluid rotation of your spine.

Lie in the Pilates rest position. Position your arms outwards on the mat, slightly below shoulder height, with the palms facing upwards. Gently engage your centre. Maintaining the neutral position of your spine and a deep connection with your centre, raise one leg at a time into the tabletop position.

Breathe in to prepare. Breathe out as you move your legs to the right (the legs and spine follow the same direction) and sequentially rotate your pelvis, lower back and mid back to the right, keeping the shoulder blades anchored on the mat. Finish by rolling your head and neck to the left, keeping the back of your neck long. Breathe in wide to the sides and back of the ribcage whilst maintaining your spinal rotation. Breathe out as you roll your head and neck to the midline and continue sequentially rolling your spine, pelvis and legs back to the midline. Repeat up to 10 times, alternating sides.

THE PROGRAMME

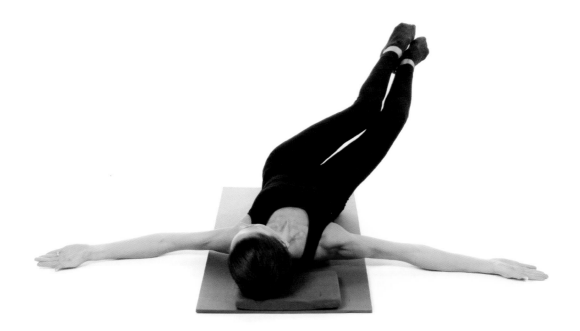

Focus on keeping your waist equally long on both sides as your spine rotates

➤ This is a precise exercise where the movement of your back is under the control of your abdominal muscles. Do not allow the weight of your legs to dictate the movement.

➤ If you feel that the movement is too challenging, modify your position to begin with. Maintaining neutral spinal alignment, position your knees closer to your chest and relax your knees to lower the heels towards your sitting bones. As your control improves, you can progress towards the true starting position.

➤ Ensure you maintain a neutral spine throughout – think of your tailbone reaching forwards towards your heels.

➤ Maintain a connection between your lower ribcage and the top of your pelvis to avoid the ribcage flaring forwards.

➤ Focus on keeping your waist equally long on both sides as your spine rotates.

the cool down

- ✓ seated hamstring stretch
- ✓ lying nerve stretch
- ✓ gluteal stretch
- ✓ cat stretch
- ✓ hip flexor stretch
- ✓ roll down

back to life
Avoid Bad Habits

Spend just 5 minutes people-watching in a busy precinct and you will observe mums rushing through town pushing baby-carriers, laden down with toddler paraphernalia, people on crutches hobbling by in unsupportive sheepskin boots or flip flops, cyclists whizzing past with all sorts of bags slung over their shoulders, shoppers overloaded with plastic bags, commuters burdened by their cases and bulging backpacks. Perhaps you can identify with someone in this picture?

Spend a moment considering the following points and you can minimise the stress you place on your body in everyday life.

- Wear supportive footwear to walk to and from work or when you know you are going to be active and on your feet for a few hours.

- Select bags that are appropriately sized and fit for purpose. If using a laptop, invest in a purpose-designed laptop bag and carry it with the strap positioned across your body. Carrying your laptop bag on one shoulder will place asymmetrical load on your spine and may trigger your pain.

- When using a backpack, ensure that you use both straps to distribute the weight evenly and pack heavier items at the back of your bag so that they are positioned closest to your spine to minimise their weight.

- Allow plenty of time to get from one place to the next to avoid frantic movement and stress.

- Investing in a great pillow will provide support to your neck and allow you a good night's sleep.

- Avoid the cycle of 'all or nothing' as described in week two.

Avoid the cycle of 'all or nothing' as described in week two. Try to avoid frantic movement and stress

WEEK FIVE Checklist:

✓ 1. I can maintain the tabletop position of my back when practising movements in four-point kneeling and do not arch my back.

✓ 2. I am avoiding common day-to-day bad habits when moving about.

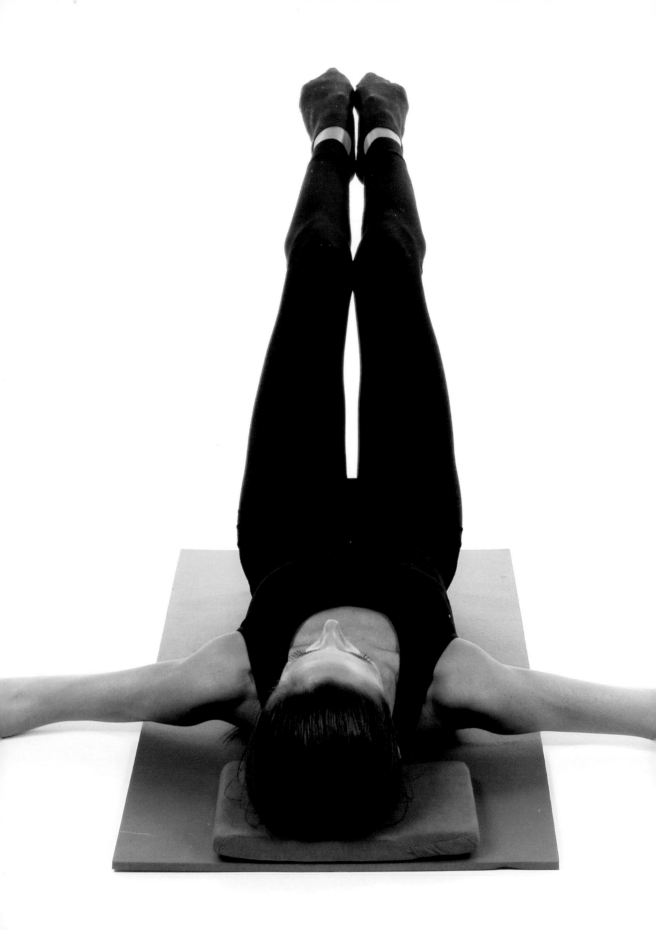

week 6

the warm up

- ✓ hundreds *level one*
- ✓ one leg stretch *level one*
- ✓ double leg stretch *level one*
- ✓ the clam *level one*
- ✓ hip twist *level one*
- ✓ shoulder bridge *level one*
- ✓ arm openings

the exercises

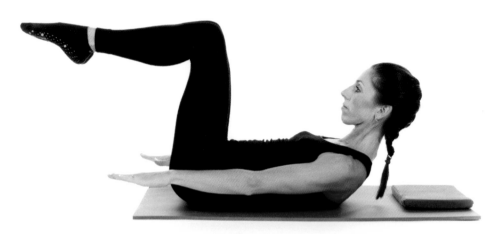

1. abdominal prep in tabletop with challenge

Trains balance and strength of the abdominal muscles to enable controlled movement of your spine and ribcage.

Lie in the Pilates rest position. Gently engage your centre. Maintaining the neutral position of your spine and a deep connection with your centre, position one leg at a time into the tabletop position.

Breathe in to prepare. Breathe out as you nod your chin and sequentially curl your head, neck, shoulders and upper back forwards while holding the tabletop position of your legs. Raise your arms to hover off the mat. Breathe in and, holding your abdominal prep position, extend your legs upwards. Breathe out and fold your legs back into the tabletop position. Breathe in as you sequentially lengthen and lower the upper body to the mat. Repeat up to 10 times.

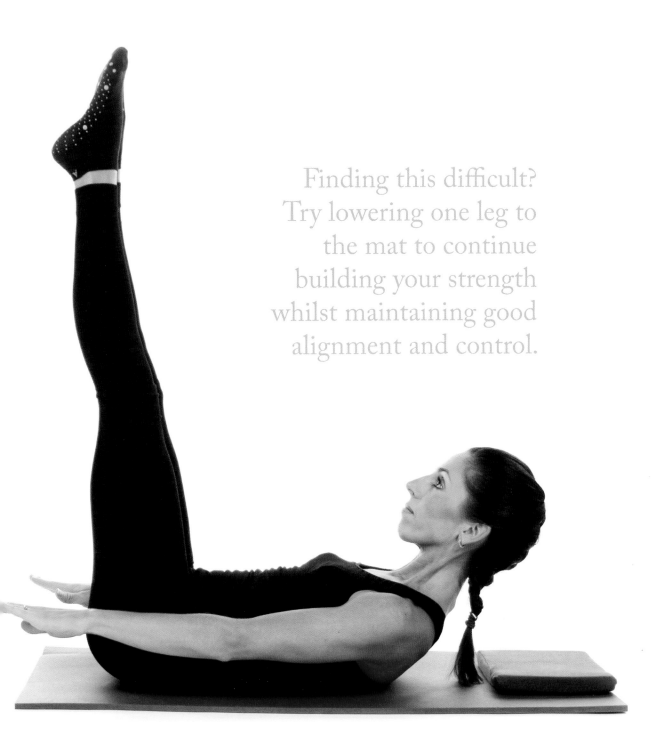

Finding this difficult?
Try lowering one leg to
the mat to continue
building your strength
whilst maintaining good
alignment and control.

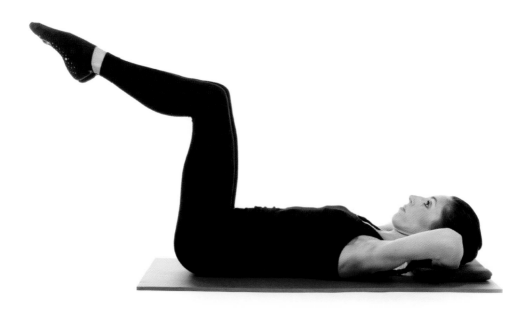

2. oblique prep in tabletop with challenge

Trains balance and strength of the abdominal muscles to enable controlled rotary movement of your spine and ribcage.

Lie in the Pilates rest position. Place your hands at the back of your head for light support. Position your elbows wide, just within your peripheral vision. Gently engage your centre. Maintaining the neutral position of your spine and a deep connection with your centre, position one leg at a time into the tabletop position.

Breathe in to prepare. Breathe out as you nod your chin and sequentially rotate your head, neck, shoulders and ribcage towards your left hip, keeping your legs lifted in the tabletop position. Breathe in and extend your right leg forwards on a diagonal. Breathe out and bend your right leg back into tabletop position. Breathe in as you sequentially lengthen and lower the upper body back to the mat back in the midline starting position, keeping your legs lifted in the tabletop position. Repeat up to 10 times, alternating sides.

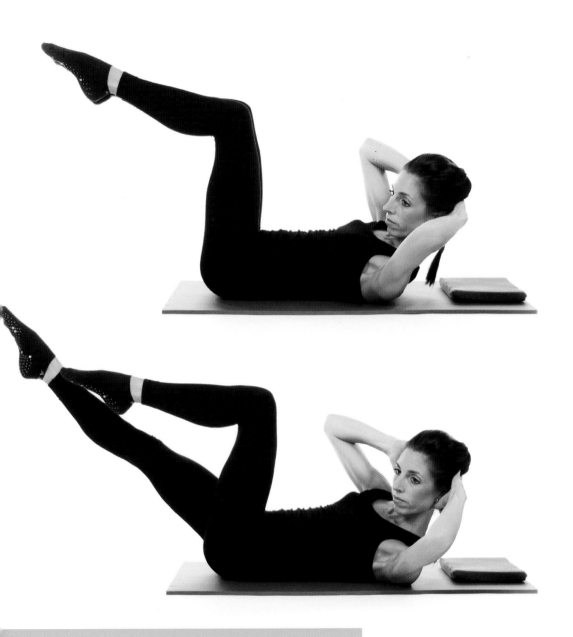

➤ Keep your trunk equally long throughout the movement to avoid any upwards hip hitching or downwards trunk tilting. There should be no shortening of your trunk on either side.

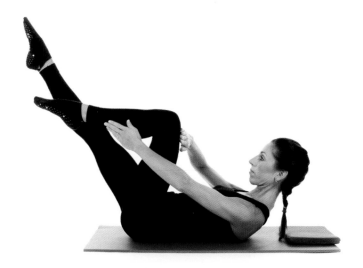

3. one leg stretch *(level five)*

Trains stability of your lower back and pelvis during coordinated movement of your legs.

Lie in the Pilates rest position. Gently engage your centre. Maintaining the neutral position of your spine and a deep connection with your centre, raise one leg at a time into the tabletop position. Then curl your head, neck, shoulders and upper body forwards into the abdominal preparation position.

Breathe in to prepare. Breathe out as you extend your right leg forwards and upwards on a diagonal line. Simultaneously reach your left hand to the outside of your left leg and place your right hand across the top of your left knee. Take a short breath in. Breathe out as you return your right leg and extend your left leg forwards and upwards on a diagonal line. Simultaneously reach your right hand to the outside of your right lower leg and place your left hand across the top of your right knee.

Continue alternating legs and arms up to 10 times, keeping the upper body lifted in the abdominal preparation position. Breathe out each time you extend your leg and take a short breath in as you alternate legs and arms. To finish, lower your upper body and then your legs to the mat one at a time.

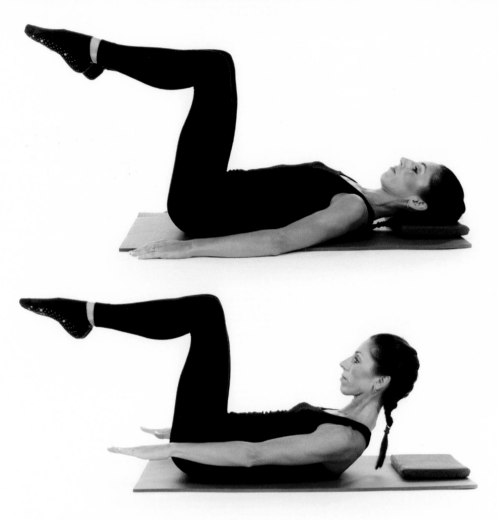

4. hundreds *(level four)*

You can further challenge your abdominal core by extending your legs forwards on a diagonal. A Pilates band looped under the soles of the feet will help to support the weight of your legs while you build the endurance required for the ultimate 100!

 ## 5. roll up see page 102

 ## 6. roll up with obliques see page 116

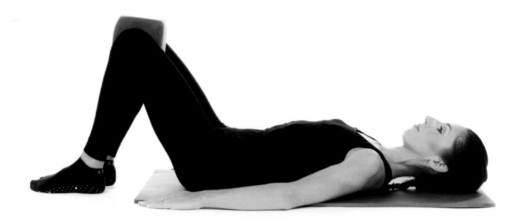

7. shoulder bridge *(level two)*

Teaches you to mobilise each joint in your back whilst strengthening key muscles to improve pelvic stability.

Lie in the Pilates rest position. To avoid any unwanted pressure through your neck, remove any pillows that you may have under your neck. Gently engage your centre. Breathe in to prepare. As you breathe out, gently roll your lower back into the mat, then float your tailbone upwards and continue to peel your spine off the mat, bone by bone, until you are resting on your shoulder blades. Breathe in and hold the shoulder bridge position.

Keeping a level pelvis, breathe out as you lift your left foot away from the mat and extend your leg forwards. Breathe in and fold your leg back into the shoulder bridge position. Repeat by lifting and extending your right leg forwards. Repeat up to 10 alternating leg reaches and then breathe out and roll down one bone at a time into the neutral spine starting position.

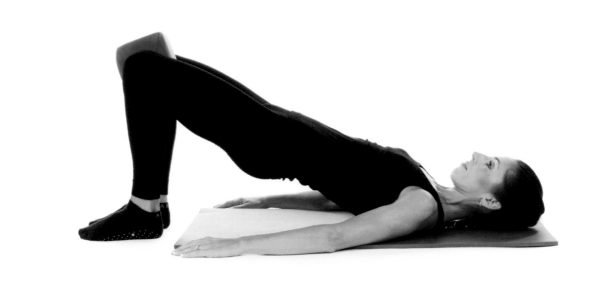

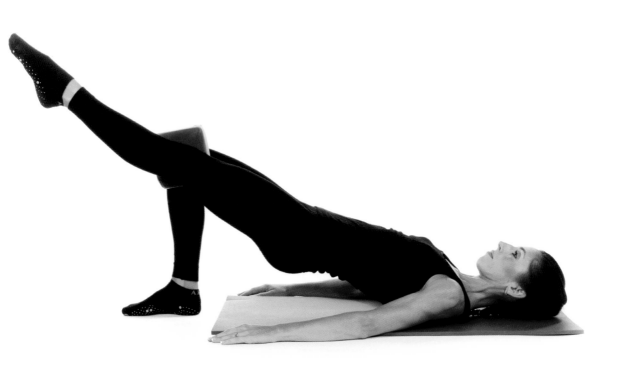

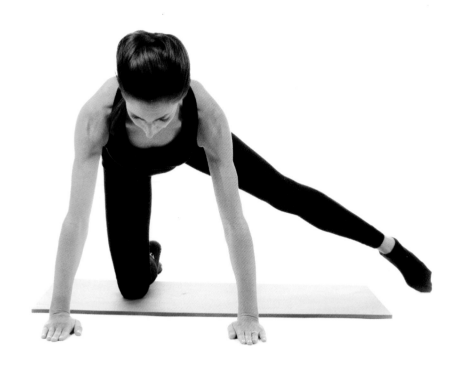

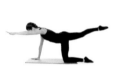 ## 8. swimming in four-point kneeling progression see page 120

9. side kick in kneeling prep

The ultimate in balance, stability and control whilst also mobilising and strengthening the hip and pelvic muscles.

Move onto all fours. Place your hands slightly forwards of your shoulders and your knees directly under your hips. Straighten your left leg and position it out to the side with your left foot in line with your left knee. Lengthen and align your spine into the neutral position. Glide your shoulder blades down your upper spine into the shape of a V. Position your head and neck in line with your trunk and lengthen the back of your neck. Gently engage your centre.

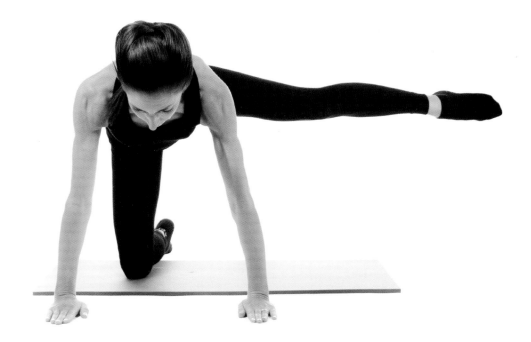

Breathe in to prepare. Breathe out as you reach and lift your left leg to hip height. Breathe in as you lower your left leg lightly to the mat. Repeat up to 10 times and then repeat on the opposite side.

HELP FROM THE PHYSIO

➤ Lacking flexibility in your hip joint? Lift your leg to hip height, start with a smaller leg lift and increase over time as your hip joint becomes more flexible.

➤ It is ideal to feel the gluteal muscles on both sides of your body working strongly throughout this exercise as your supporting hip muscles are also working hard.

➤ Your shoulders and hips should be facing downwards to avoid unwanted rotation of your pelvis or upper body.

➤ Focus on keeping your waist equally long on both sides.

➤ Avoid sinking down into your supporting shoulders and ribcage. Think of lifting your shoulders away from your hand and your ribcage upwards from the mat.

➤ Lengthen the back of the neck throughout and keep the head and neck lifted.

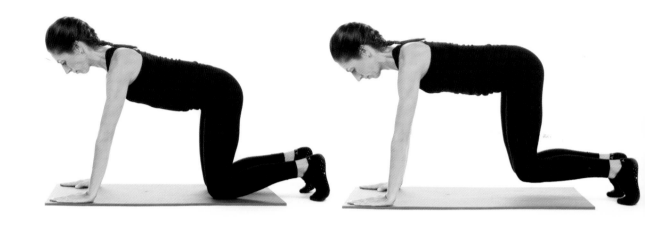

10. leg pull in prone prep

A strength and stability challenge for the upper and lower body, which commands total body awareness and integration.

Kneel on all fours with hands slightly forward of your shoulders and knees directly under your hips. Curl the balls of your feet underneath you. Lengthen and align your spine into the neutral position. Position your head and neck in line with your trunk. Keep arms straight and gently lift your chest away from the mat to stabilise your shoulder blades. Gently engage your centre.

Breathe in to prepare. Breathe out as you lift and hover your knees away from the mat, maintaining the shape of your four-point kneeling. Breathe in wide and hold this position. Breathe out as you lower your knees to the mat. Repeat up to 10 times.

If your wrists feel sore, try making a fist and supporting your body on your fists and not on your palms.

THE PROGRAMME

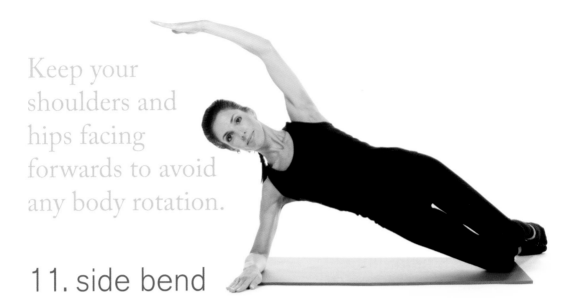

Keep your
shoulders and
hips facing
forwards to avoid
any body rotation.

11. side bend

Creates a stretch for the side of the body, lateral
mobilisation of the spine and stabilisation of the
shoulder complex.

Lie on your side on the mat, supported on your underside elbow and
forearm. Bend your knees slightly. Stack your shoulders, hips, knees and
feet. Lengthen your uppermost arm along the upper side of your trunk and
thigh. Align your neck and head to follow the line created by your trunk and
lengthen the back of your neck. Create a small lift from your supporting
shoulder and underside ribcage to avoid sinking towards the mat. Gently
engage your centre.

Breathe in to prepare. Breathe out as you lift your pelvis and ribcage away
from the mat to create a side bend of your trunk. Reach your uppermost
arm overhead and slightly forwards into your peripheral vision. Breathe in
wide to the uppermost side of your ribcage to encourage lateral expansion
of the ribcage. Breathe out as you lower your pelvis to the mat, controlling
the placement of your underside ribcage and shoulder blade. Repeat up to
10 times on each side.

the cool down

✓ seated hamstring stretch
✓ lying nerve stretch
✓ gluteal stretch
✓ cat stretch
✓ hip flexor stretch
✓ roll down

back to life
Get Active

To maintain good health, spend 30 minutes, at least five days a week, carrying out moderate intensity exercise. Pilates is a great form of exercise to improve muscle tone and balance, alignment and movement control. However, unlike cardiovascular exercise, it does not exercise your heart and lungs or burn fat.

Why not step up a gear in your everyday life? Start walking or cycling instead of taking the car for short journeys. Use the stairs instead of taking the lift and think about more manual activities to enjoy such as gardening.

- Walking at a medium to fast pace improves cardiovascular fitness as well as muscle strength. Remember to wear supportive footwear, use your Pilates centre for support and take a friend to make it fun.

- Swimming is also great for exercising your upper and lower body as well as challenging your heart and lungs. If unsure of your technique, it is worth checking in with a coach who can advise you on ways to make your swimming most efficient. Like any form of exercise, pace yourself and set realistic goals.

- Cycling also works the arms and legs whilst still being fun. Wear a helmet and cycling shorts for safety and comfort and always stretch your thighs afterwards.

WALKING at a medium to fast pace improves cardiovascular fitness as well as muscle strength. Pace yourself and set realistic goals.

WEEK SIX Checklist:

✓ **1.** Now that I have worked my way through the programme, I can easily find my neutral spine and set my centre in any position

✓ **2.** I am moving about with better posture, ease and confidence.

✓ **3.** I am generally more active and mentally focused on how my body is moving

Index

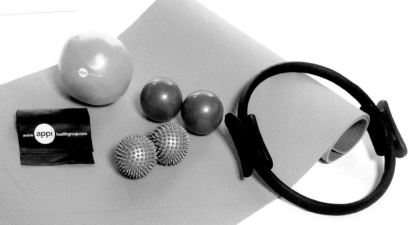
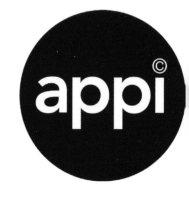

If you are interested in any of the products featured in this book, you can order them through our website www.appihealthgroup.com. APPI products are of the highest quality and are designed by APPI physiotherapists for use in clinic, in the studio or at home.

OUR 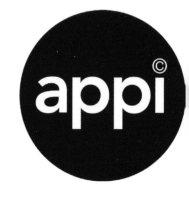 RANGE INCLUDES:

- **THE APPI SOCK**

A clinically designed Pilates sock with capturing grip points and unique reflexology points. Ideal for use in Pilates or simply round the house; use them to ensure a safe and non-slippery work out. One size fits all.

- **THE PILATES MAT**

The first Pilates mat specifically designed for studio and home use by industry experts, the new, all-purpose length (60cm x 140cm x 6mm), non-slip under surface and exercise-specific top surface offer maximum support and comfort.

- **PILATES SITTING BLOCK**

The Pilates sitting block (30cm x 20cm x 5cm) will be invaluable in many Pilates movements. Designed to support the body in sitting postures and ideal for anyone with lower back pain.

- **SPIKY MASSAGE BALLS**

These 9cm balls can be used to massage the feet, elongate and release tight muscles and provide self-massage for the trapezius and lower back muscles. A great help in Pilates when you need to focus on strengthening without bracing other muscles.

- **PILATES BAND**

The Pilates band is a versatile product for exercise, rehabilitation and conditioning. Available in lighter resistance for the upper body and heavier for the lower body, it is the perfect aid to keeping arms and legs beautifully toned.

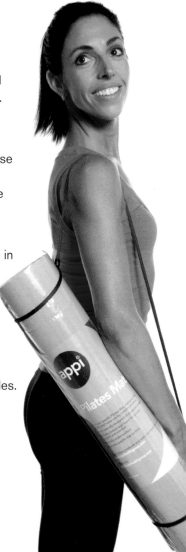